Cystitis: The new approach

Defines the causes and precipitating factors of cystitis, outlines who it affects and why, and offers a comprehensive guide to supplementary or alternative treatments.

Cystitis
The
new approach

Take positive steps towards freedom from
discomfort with a personal self-help plan

by

Dr Caroline Shreeve
M.B., B.S.(Lond.)

THORSONS PUBLISHING GROUP
Wellingborough, Northamptonshire

—————— • ——————

Rochester, Vermont

First published 1986

British Library Cataloguing in Publication Data

Shreeve, Caroline
Cystitis: the new approach.
1. Bladder — Inflammation — Treatment
2. Self-care, Health
I. Title
616.6'2306   RG485.C9

ISBN 0-7225-1226-0

Printed and bound in Great Britain

CONTENTS

Introduction

Why another book about cystitis? For years, there was little lay information on the subject, and then – as was the case with the premenstrual syndrome (PMS) magazine features and books on the subject began to appear in profusion. Many of these have provided women with much needed information, and have helped to boost their confidence in a situation in which it is often difficult to feel any hope at all.

Knowing more about their disorder has had the special benefit of enabling women to cope with recurrent cystitis attacks, and often to end them, without visiting their doctors or taking drugs.

Still further need exists, though, for informative books on the subject. Cystitis is one of those complaints about which most patients know almost as much as their doctors. Although medical science has made some marvellous advances over the last decade, particularly in the fields of microsurgery, organ transplantation and *in-vitro* fertilization, little of note has been achieved in the field of cystitis research. *Why* certain women suffer attack after attack and others remain free of it, and *why* symptoms continue in the absence of infected urine, are questions that have continued to baffle both GPs and urological specialists. And because doctors frequently fail to cure their cystitis patients, they are criticized for being ignorant and uncaring.

Patients, on the other hand, many of whom turn up for further advice and treatment every two or three months, are regarded sometimes – regrettably – as hypochondriac, and told that there is nothing further that can be done for them. This is not only very poor psychology, but it is also untrue, since a great deal can be done to help individual sufferers to identify the causes of their attacks and work out ways of avoiding them.

An admission of defeat on behalf of orthodox medicine is only a poor half of the story. There are a number of disorders for which alternative therapies provide more effective treatment than conventional medicine. And when antibiotics are no longer effective, or not indicated, then we doctors would do well to discuss alternative forms of treatment with our patients.

Slowly, of course, the gap between the GP or hospital doctor and the 'alternative' practitioner is narrowing. While ten years ago many orthodox doctors were suspicious of, for example, osteopaths and chiropractors, and attached little credence to homoeopathy or hypnotherapy, it is not at all unusual nowadays for them to refer their patients to such therapists, for complementary or alternative treatment.

Certainly most cystitis sufferers would agree that the more guns brought to bear on the problem, the better. You have to have experienced this complaint to know of the pain, distress and inconvenience it can cause. In addition, there is the embarrassment many women feel about the amount of time they take off work and the necessity of explaining, yet again, to an incredulous employer that yet another attack has started.

There are many women in this unenviable position, however. If you, the reader, are one of them, it may offer you some consolation to know that you are not alone, or in any sense 'peculiar'. Just as backache, digestive upsets and infections of the upper respiratory tract (nasal membranes, throat, tonsils) are among the commonest general problems a GP sees in his daily surgery, cystitis is one of the most common – if not *the* commonest complaint – affecting women. In any one year, about 1.7 million women suffer from cystitis, and many of them get an average of four to five attacks in twelve months.

I mentioned the embarrassment that cystitis can cause to working women, in terms of time off work and having to explain to employers and colleagues. With the sexual liberation that has taken place since the sixties, you may not think that cystitis could possibly present any cause for embarrassment. But some people still shy away from the word, as though it were a secret female disorder to be discussed in the same breath as labour pains, period problems and a discharge 'down below'. Others – including many women who have never experienced it – find it hard to believe that a minor bladder complaint could possibly be responsible for such distress. Women are often the most severe critics of their own sex, and I have seen shop assistant cystitis sufferers in their late teens and twenties threatened with 'the sack' by their female supervisor if they took any more time off work for a 'trivial complaint'.

This attitude, wherever it is encountered, only makes life more difficult. As we are becoming increasingly aware, stress has a significant role to play in the generation of many medical conditions. And anxiety and tension can only serve in such a situation to increase the misery and pain.

I am not implying that a difficult boss and fear of being out of work are responsible for attacks of cystitis as such. What I am suggesting is that inner tension, stress and worry are reflected in the condition of our bodies, and how they react to harmful stimuli. It is believed that prolonged emotional or physical stress decreases the power of our immune defence systems to ward off invading bacteria and viruses, making us far more vulnerable to infection. There is also no doubt whatever that inner conflict and worry lower our pain threshold, making us more susceptible to the effects of pain from any source.

Working women are not alone in suffering from the handicaps associated with recurrent cystitis. Having to cope at home with babies and toddlers, taking older children to school, packing school (and perhaps work) lunches, visiting the supermarket and the laundrette, and seeing that the dog gets his daily run round the park can become an almost intolerable burden when you are feverish, in pain, and forever needing to spend a penny.

Even arrangements normally made for pleasure, such as an appointment with your hairdresser, a coffee morning with neighbours, or clothes shopping with a friend, lose all attraction when your bladder demands your full attention. Even to your nearest and dearest, you can start to become a drag. Husbands and children are nearly always understanding and sympathetic at first. But when you complain of the symptoms time and time again, and there is nothing they can actually do to make you feel better, then your symptoms frustrate them as much as they do you. This is especially true when these symptoms prevent you from going out on promised treats and trips.

The main problem – as it is with so many recurrent conditions such as backache and period pains – is that there is little to *see*! You can produce no fracture plasters, vivid purple bruises, dramatic rashes or startling X-ray results. All your family sees is you wrapped round a hot water bottle, drinking pints of water, and unable to join in with normal family activities. Certainly, you may be passing pink coloured or even crimson urine. But few sufferers drag their family members into the bathroom to examine the latest specimen they have produced, or wave a thermometer at them to indicate a mild temperature rise. So although they may not actually suffer in silence, many cystitis sufferers find that they end up suffering alone.

The first step in overcoming these problems is to understand all the relevant facts that have been gathered about cystitis, its causes, and its treatment. Many women *do* in fact 'suffer in silence' at least with respect to their doctors, since once they have been told that no further medication or investigations are likely to prove worthwhile, they understandably get deterred from repeated visits to the surgery.

What is really required is a clear idea of what is happening inside the bladder to cause cystitis symptoms, of when to visit your GP with a specimen of urine and a request for treatment, and when it is quite safe to manage one's 'water problems' by oneself. It is also essential to know about the numerous factors that can cause, or at least trigger, a cystitis attack; to find out what is causing these attacks in *your* particular case; and what preventative measures are available.

The rest of this book sets out this information in simple, straightforward terms, and discusses the natural means available for treating the condition, either independently from conventional methods or as adjuncts to it. It should give renewed hope and encouragement to even the most chronic cystitis sufferer.

1

Defining Cystitis

In order to understand cystitis properly, it is a good idea to know a little about the bladder and its connections with both the ureters (urine tubes) and kidneys above, and the urine outlet tube (urethra) below. This is important, since although the word 'cystitis' refers simply to an inflamed urinary bladder, this organ – like all others – clearly does not exist or function in isolation! It is an inseparable part of the body's urine excretion system, and infection within the bladder can spread up the ureters, if left untreated, and cause a serious infection within the kidneys.

The urethra's structure and function are also important in this context. It is the area where much of the pain associated with cystitis is felt, and its lower opening where urine is voided is in contact with the body's immediate external environment. This accessibility to the exterior makes it the focal point of many irritants now known to be responsible, possibly for true cystitis attacks, and certainly for attacks of 'urethritis' or the 'urethral syndrome'. The urethra's proximity to the exterior also provides us with a chance to apply first-aid remedies and preventive measures directly.

Structure
The bladder is a hollow sac or reservoir for holding urine, and it lies in the pelvis, in front of the womb (uterus) in a woman, and in front of the lower end of the large bowel (rectum) in a man. It lies immediately behind the pubic bone which you can feel as a hard, bony projection in a direct line downwards from your navel. The bladder projects up into the lower abdomen when full, as a rounded dome. When empty, however, it is about the size of a

large fist and more or less pyramidal in shape. It receives a steady dribble of urine from the kidneys, which are situated higher up in the abdominal cavity, one on either side of the spine.

The kidneys are protected by a special kind of fat in which they are embedded, and also by the muscles around the spine and by the lower ribs. The term 'floating kidney' refers to the looseness of the kidney's attachments when a great deal of body fat, including some of that surrounding the kidneys, has been lost. On the top or 'pole' of each kidney sits an adrenal gland, responsible for producing several vital hormones. These include adrenaline and noradrenaline which we release in response to stress.

Between the kidneys runs the aorta, the body's largest artery, from which they receive their blood supply by means of its renal branches. Also lying between the kidneys is the inferior vena cava, a large vein draining all the abdominal and pelvic organs – including the kidneys and bladder – of used blood, which it returns to the heart and lungs.

The urine made in the kidneys reaches the bladder by means of two tubes, the ureters, which open into the back of the bladder on each side. Each opening is guarded by a valve which under normal conditions prevents backflow of stored urine up the ureters and into the kidneys. As the bladder fills up, the muscle of which its wall is composed (the 'detrusor' muscle), unfolds and adapts itself to provide a larger capacity. The muscle fibres are not stretched when the bladder contains only a small amount of urine, which is why, under normal conditions, we do not have a perpetual feeling of wanting to pass urine.

The pressure inside does start to rise, though, once the volume of urine within has reached a certain point. It is then that the 'stretch receptor' cells (special nerve cells) in the bladder lining become activated, and we start to become aware of needing to open our bladders. There is a certain amount of individual variation in bladder capacity; but most of us seem to empty our bladder when it contains around half a pint of urine. Generally, about a pint can be stored before severe discomfort is experienced.

Urine passes out of the bladder through the urethra. This is a muscular tube with two valves (or sphincters) which guard its point of exit from the bladder, and its lower end from which urine is discharged. Both of these valves control the urine's outflow.

In a man, the urethra is relatively long (between 7 and 8 in) and passes down through the substance of the prostate gland before turning forwards and running the length of the penis to the exterior. In a woman, the urethra is much shorter (about 1½ in), and it opens directly into the anogenital area immediately in front of the vagina. Because of these anatomical differences, the risk of germs (bacteria) passing from the anus (lower end of the rectum) into the urethra and up into the bladder is very much greater in a woman. This goes part of the way to explaining why cystitis is much more common in the female sex.

Urine is discharged from the bladder by reflex action in a baby who has not yet learned bladder control. Older children and adults learn to override this reflex and wait until it is convenient to pass urine. This then takes place by allowing the bladder wall muscle to contract.

The inner layer of the bladder is mucous membrane, which is loose in texture and thrown into folds which open out when the bladder wall is stretched. The membrane itself is lined with a delicate tissue, the 'epithelium'. The interior of the bladder is richly supplied with both blood vessels and nerves, and can be viewed by means of cystoscope. This is the lighted instrument introduced up the urethra and into the bladder under sedation or general anaesthetic by urological surgeons when they investigate urinary problems.

The nervous supply to the bladder permits sensations of both pain and bladder distension to be experienced. It also affords the means by which the bladder is opened reflexly when full, in a baby, and by which it is controlled by the conscious mind of an older child or adult until release is convenient.

Birth defects affecting the lower end of the spinal cord (for example, spina bifida), spinal cord injuries, and certain disorders of the central nervous system (such as multiple sclerosis), can interfere with conscious control of the bladder's function and result in incontinence.

Inflammation

It is easier to understand *why* cystitis hurts so much, if we understand first what happens when tissues become inflamed.

The four characteristics of acute inflammation wherever it

occurs in the body, are redness, increased heat, swelling and pain, and they are due to the cellular activity that takes place in the affected tissues. The factors capable of causing inflammation are numerous, two important ones being tissue injury and the presence of irritating chemical substances.

Whatever the trigger factor to a state of inflammation, the result is the release of the chemical histamine from the damaged cells. Histamine is also the cell chemical which is released during the course of an allergic reaction and, in a number of respects, allergy and inflammation are similar processes. Histamine causes the small blood vessels (capillaries) in the neighbourhood of the irritant both to expand and to leak.

The fact that the capillaries expand, increasing the supply of blood to the area, accounts for the redness and increased temperature that occur in inflammation. The leaking of fluid and protein from the blood out through the capillary walls and into the surrounding tissue spaces is responsible for the swelling. The pain is due to two factors. One of these is irritation of the nerve endings by the chemical substances involved in the inflammatory process, and the other is pressure resulting from the local accumulation of tissue fluid.

The escaped tissue fluid fulfils a very useful purpose. It has a slightly antiseptic effect, and it also dilutes the concentration of irritating chemical compounds derived either from the exterior (as in an insect sting) or from the damaged cells themselves. The white cells from the blood enter the inflamed area and join forces with other white cells already present to engulf and destroy foreign particles, including bacteria and dead tissue cells.

When the inflammatory process, which like the immune defence system is one of the body's main defence mechanisms, is successful, adhesions form as the tissue fluid and its proteins form a clot, and new tissue grows into the area. Initially this consists of new blood vessels and fibrous connective tissue. Some tissues are able to reform themselves following damage; but others, such as muscle and nerve cells, cannot do so.

The lining of the bladder and urethra is able to effect a reasonably good repair operation. But scar tissue forms as well, and fissures (small cracks) appear which bleed, heal over with scar tissue between attacks, and reopen to bleed again on subsequent occasions.

Everyone is familiar with the appearance of inflamed skin around a cut, or in the vicinity of a burn or infected spots. Such areas of inflammation remind us continually of their presence and, when they exist in areas of the body which can be seen, we make every effort we can to protect the affected area from further damage.

Such precautions are a great deal more difficult to take when the inflamed surface is inside. Anyone who suffers from a peptic ulcer will be aware of the acute pain that ensues when excess hydrochloric acid is secreted by the stomach lining on to the raw, inflamed area. In many people, the slightest dietary indiscretion will cause very severe pain, and it is necessary to take either regular doses of an alkaline preparation to neutralize stomach acidity (i.e. 'antacids', like aluminium hydroxide gel – Aludrox) or a drug which antagonizes the effect of the free acid particles on the ulcer site (such as cimetidine – Tagomet, or ranitidine – Zantac).

Symptoms

In the case of the bladder, the inflamed, tender lining is in constant contact with urine, which is usually acidic, and sometimes highly so. The urethral lining is usually the first to become inflamed, and as it is continuous with the lining of the bladder, the inflammatory process sometimes spreads throughout both of these organs.

Quite often, however, the bladder lining remains unaffected and what is called cystitis is in fact inflammation confined to the lining of the urethra ('urethritis', or the 'urethral syndrome'). When the infection is confined 'down below' and does not involve ureters or kidneys, then the symptoms of 'urethritis' and of 'cystitis proper' are indistinguishable from one another and recognizable immediately by all who have ever suffered an attack of either in the past. They include:

* a painful, burning sensation on passing urine;
* 'urgency', which is the great and immediate need to get to the toilet to pass urine – which often then consists of only a drop or two;
* pains in the lower abdomen and lower back;
* nausea and occasionally vomiting;
* dark, sometimes bad-smelling urine that may have a pinkish colour or obviously contain bright red blood;

* getting up at night to pass urine;
* a very painful burning feeling in the urethral outlet which can radiate as far as the vaginal lips.

There is an important difference between cystitis (I will use that name both for bladder and for urethral inflammation from now onwards, except when it is necessary to differentiate between them), however, and a disorder such as tonsillitis, or chickenpox. These last-mentioned are infections that *involve* inflammation, but which can unarguably be attributed in each case to an invading bacteria or virus. Cystitis, by way of contrast, is by definition simply a state of inflammation, and as we have seen, inflammation has a wide variety of possible causes. Many people regard cystitis – wrongly – as an infection of the bladder.

But bacterial infection is only one of a number of possible causes for cystitis. Cystitis is in fact a sign, a message from the body that all is not as it should be, and an indication that an underlying irritant – maybe a bacteria – should be sought.

Causes
The numerous non-infective causes of cystitis account in most cases for the negative results that are returned time after time from hospital laboratories all over the country. This can prove very frustrating if you have pinned your hopes on a prescription for antibiotics to solve your problem.

Your GP is quite right in asking for a urine specimen, and requesting the tests known as 'culture and sensitivity' from the hospital's pathology department. As mentioned above, untreated infection in the bladder can ascend the ureters and reach the kidneys, producing a serious kidney infection. What is less commendable is the habit a few doctors have of handing out antibiotic prescriptions time after time upon request, without examining the patient, or carrying out any investigations. Once thought to be even less commendable than that, because less rational, was the prescribing of antibiotics anyway, even in the face of a negative bacteriological result.

It is now realized that, since the urethra is so closely associated anatomically with the vagina, organisms from the latter are prone to infect it periodically. When this happens, the bacteria may not be apparent on urine culture, but it is thought to be wise to prescribe antibiotics all the same.[1]

Bacteria

The bacteria found in infected urine are nearly always the same as those that are normally present around the anus and in the faeces (motions). The commonest variety is Escherichia coli (E. coli for short). The external opening of the urethra is only a couple of inches away from the anus, and it is possible to give the bacteria in that region a helping hand to reach and travel up the urethra without being aware of doing so. These are the means by which this may be done:

* incorrect use of toilet paper. The correct direction in which to use toilet paper is from front to back, although most people seem to have an inborn tendency to 'wipe' in the other direction, judging by the comments patients often make to this particular piece of advice. Used in the way I suggest, there is far less danger of the toilet paper acting as a free vehicle of transport from the anus and motions to the urethral opening.

* sexual intercourse. Cystitis used to be called the 'honeymoon disease' and 'honeymoon cystitis' is still referred to sometimes. Lovemaking can, like toilet paper, contribute towards infective cystitis by the male partner's fingers or penis transferring bacteria forwards from the perianal region (skin around the anus) to the urethral opening. This factor is less easy to control if you are married or have a regular sexual partner, as the last thing you want to introduce into a fulfilling sex life is inhibition or unnecessary restraint. All the same, certain tips are worth passing on.

First, discuss the matter with your husband or boyfriend and explain what you are trying to avoid, i.e. contaminating your urethral opening with faecal bacteria. If you are a chronic cystitis sufferer, your sex life may well have been less than fulfilling recently anyway, so it is likely that you will get co-operation on this point. Ask him to avoid touching your anal region, and then your vaginal region with his fingertips, and also, if possible, to avoid sliding the tip of his penis down between your thighs to the region of your anus, and then lifting it upwards with a dragging movement to enter your vagina. This is bound to transfer any bacteria in the region to the entrance of your urethra.

Take the added precaution yourself, of washing and drying your anal region and your perineum (area between vagina and anus) before love-making sessions. Use unscented soap, warm, not hot, water, and pat dry with clean cotton wool. Pass urine straight after a love-making session (this helps to wash out any invading bacteria that may have reached your urethra), and soap and dry the perineal area once more.

This may all sound very fiddly and a real nuisance. But it is not nearly as bothersome as an attack of infective cystitis, and soon becomes a matter of habit.

* poor hygiene. None of us likes to think that we do not pay enough attention to personal hygiene. But it is easy enough to put off a bath or an all-over wash when you are tired or the bathroom is draughty. Unfortunately, an unwashed perineal area, with a build-up of stale sweat, tiny smears of faeces and daily dust and dirt, together with minute fragments of soft toilet paper and a few dead skin cells and pubertal hairs is just the breeding ground for faecal bacteria.

The conditions are made even more conducive to their welfare if you wear nylon panties and tights, and tight jeans. These keep the area sweaty, moist and warm. The best approach, therefore, is to wash daily – in or out of the bath – with plain, unscented soap, and also straight after passing a motion. Angela Kilmartin, in her useful book: *Cystitis – A Complete Self-Help Guide*, suggests washing the anal region with cold, boiled water, which can be done by pouring it from a bottle on to the anal region after using the paper as described above.

The water can be poured over the urethral region as you sit on the toilet seat and lean back slightly. The water then trickles down over the vaginal lips and the anus, which can then be patted dry with cotton wool.

You can carry out this routine quite easily when travelling, or away from home. Take a small plastic bottle of boiled water with you, safely done up with a screw top, and a small plastic bag containing some clean cotton wool. You can also take a tiny piece of unscented soap with you in a piece of greaseproof paper or clingfilm, if you are not sure of finding suitable soap for the purpose wherever you are going to visit.

* the use of vaginal tampons. The string of tampons can easily transfer bacteria from the anal region to the urethral opening. If you have used tampons for years instead of sanitary towels, you may not like the thought of going back to the latter. All the same, my advice is to avoid tampons at all costs, at least until you have been free of cystitis attacks for a whole year, and if and when you *do* return to them, pay even greater attention to personal hygiene than before.

In case it is years since you have used sanitary towels, and have not kept up with recent developments in that field, I can assure you that considerable advances have been made in their design, and that they do not involve your wearing the same barbaric monthly apparel which was once necessary.

Sanitary belts, with a string fore and aft bearing an enamelled metal hook device, can safely be relegated to the Curiosities Museum. Sanitary towels are slimmer and more streamlined, are kept in position by a press-on technique, and come individually packaged in attractively designed plastic wrapping (Nana, by Peaudouce, are, in my opinion, the most appealing).

Try also to avoid wearing nylon panties and tights, and tight trousers and jeans. These increase the amount of sweat you form in the genital region, and keep the area hot and clammy because there is no means by which the perspiration can escape. Choose open-crotch tights, or old-fashioned stockings and suspender belt if you happen to like them. Go also for skirts and dresses rather than trousers, and replace nylon or synthetic fibre underwear with pure cotton.

Non-infective irritants

Women who suffer from recurrent attacks of non-bacterial cystitis are thought to have unusually sensitive epithelial linings to their bladders and urethras. It is also thought that in many women, urethritis rather than cystitis is the basic, underlying cause. Bouts of inflammation of the urethral lining are likely to be triggered by any of the following:

* contraceptive devices. It seems that being on the Pill may slightly increase your chances of cystitis attacks. The use of spermicidal cream can irritate the urethra if it is smeared on to the external urethral opening; and there is also a higher incidence of bladder and urethral inflammation in women who use the cap or diaphragm, or whose partners use the sheath.

* vibration. Prolonged vibration can spark off an attack. The source of vibration may be a badly sprung car seat, a rickety bicycle, a tractor seat, or the use of a vibrator on or sufficiently close to the clitoris for the urethra to be affected.

* foreign bodies in the urethra. These may be particles of dirt or dust, inadvertently transferred to the urethral opening by your lover's hands and fingernails during love-making. They may be bits of grit, fragments of straw dust, pollen or soil, or sand from the beach, following a love-making session in the open country or while camping.

Another, less common variety of foreign body is the type a number of women deliberately introduce into their urethral opening as a source of sexual pleasure. There is no field like that of sexual preference for demonstrating the possible range of human imagination and inventiveness, and some women find that stimulation of the external urethral opening brings them to the point of orgasm very quickly. Consequently, they either introduce a suitably small, preferably blunt, object into this opening during a masturbatory session, or teach their partners how to do it for them.

I do strongly advise against this practice. I am saying this neither on the grounds of sexual decency (which does not really enter into the matter), nor of aestheticism. My attitude to these affairs is very much: 'Chacun à son gout'. Simply, from the medical point of view, pushing a matchstick or biro refill tip into your urethral opening is highly likely to cause some structural damage, practically bound to introduce infection sooner or later, and may result in an exploratory search in Casualty to remove an object that has gone too far up.

Women who do this, may also find that their ability to 'hold' their urine when their bladder gets very full, becomes seriously affected, since interfering with this area can destroy the delicate valve mechanism upon which continence partly depends.

* excessive heat or cold. Just as sitting on radiators or solid fuel stoves can encourage piles (haemorrhoids) to form, and irritate existing ones, so it can bring on the symptoms of urethritis or cystitis by aggravating the sensitive lining membranes of bladder and urethra. This may come as a surprise, for many people think that it is only a chill on the bladder, from sitting on something cold and damp, which can bring on cystitis.

    Extreme cold can, of course, do this just as well as abnormally high temperatures applied to the area. Sitting down on pavements, stone walls, even on a draughty lino floor at home can provide the necessary trigger, as can (in some women) wearing cold, damp underwear, or the lower half of a swimming costume while it remains wet.

* chemical irritants. This class of cystitis causes includes some otherwise pleasant synthetic preparations you may well use daily, without imagining that they may be responsible for your repeated attacks of cystitis. Examples are perfumed soap, bath crystals, bath oils, bubble bath liquid, shampoo (if you wash your hair in the bath), talcum powder – especially the scented variety, vaginal deodorants and vaginal 'freshener' tissues.

    Swimming in a chlorinated swimming pool, adding antiseptic liquid to your own bath water (perhaps for skin trouble), and using biological washing powders for your panties, can all stimulate an oversensitive urethral and bladder lining and make it inflamed.

* food irritants and allergies. Certain spicy foods can induce cystitis attacks in some people. Likely ones are pepper, chilli powder and fresh chillis, citrus fruit, pickles containing vinegar, food marinated in vinegar or wine, large quantities of wine or acid fruit juice, and certain curry spices. Eating large quantities of chocolate can produce symptoms in some cystitis sufferers.

    Food allergies that can do this include certain proteins in cereals, beans and onions; gluten; starch and lactose (milk sugar).

* liquid intake. Drinking too little water to replace that lost by the body, results in the production of relatively small volumes of

highly concentrated urine. This can irritate the bladder and urethral lining, and is, of course, especially likely to happen in hot weather when a larger amount of fluid than usual is being lost as perspiration.

What you drink can also affect a sensitive bladder. Besides the wine mentioned above, large amounts of any type of alcohol can trigger symptoms, as can glass after glass of cola drinks, and mug upon mug of strong tea or coffee.

These are the factors, bacterial and non-infective, which can be responsible for many recurrent attacks of cystitis. Whatever the cause in *your* case, it is vital to determine, in the first instance, whether or not bacteria are involved. Much of the advice you will read in this book is of the self-help and preventive variety, and much, too, deals with the treatments that the alternative therapies have to offer.

First, though, we will take a look at the methods orthodox medicine uses to investigate a case of cystitis, including the laboratory tests on a urine sample, and how such a sample should be taken.

2

Diagnosis

Thorough investigation of recurrent cystitis is essential. In the first place it is necessary to establish that the disorder *is* cystitis, and not another disorder producing similar symptoms. Infections of the cervix and vagina can mimic cystitis and urethritis, and cause pain on passing urine, but they are also likely to produce irritation and soreness around the vaginal entrance, and a vaginal discharge.

It can be difficult, in fact, to tell just which part of you 'down below' is actually hurting. But the pain of vaginitis and cervicitis is more external and a bit further back, and usually involves the outer vaginal lips (labia). The pain you experience on passing urine in this case is due to the hot, acid urine running over the sore and inflamed labia. The urination pain of cystitis and urethritis is a little higher up inside, and nearer to the front of your genital area, close to and behind your clitoris.

Sometimes infection of the vagina and/or cervix will be found together with urethritis and possibly cystitis as well. If you are experiencing symptoms you believe add up to cystitis for the first time, or get recurrent bouts of cystitis that do not respond to self-help measures, go and see your doctor and ask for a sample of your urine to be sent for bacteriological tests.

Even though all tests in the past have proved negative, you must act promptly if you believe you may have an infection. Whether you decide to combine self-help measures with your doctor's treatment, or to consult an alternative practitioner in future, is entirely up to you. But an established infection, either in the bladder and urethra, or within the vagina and cervix, needs to be identified and treated without delay.

The second reason why recurrent cystitis needs to be investigated, particularly when infection is present yet unresponsive to treatment, is to rule out unusual predisposing causes for the attacks. These include:

* a source of infection above the bladder, for instance pyelo-nephritis associated with kidney stones;
* obstruction below the bladder, such as urethral stricture (narrowing) in a woman; either this, or a tumour, benign or malignant, in the prostate gland, may affect a man;
* a tumour or a foreign body in the bladder, which may be either a bladder stone or an object that has been pushed up through the urethra for sexual gratification (see page 20);
* spread of inflammation to the bladder from an adjacent organ, such as the colon (large bowel) or pelvic organs;
* the presence of an anatomical defect, such as a cystocoele or urethrocoele (blind pouch projecting from either the bladder or the urethra), and harbouring bacteria.

Lastly, the bacteria causing recurrent infection may simply be resistant to the antibiotic drug(s) chosen for treatment.

Doctors, especially GPs, are often severely criticized for the way they handle patients complaining of recurrent urinary problems. Like thrush infection, cystitis can be highly frustrating to treat, both from the doctor's viewpoint, and even more so, of course, from the patient's. Resistant infections, and cystitis symptoms arising for no apparent cause, *are* difficult to advise about, unless an 'all round' approach is adopted, which looks at the patient's lifestyle for causes associated with stress, diet, exercise and contact with synthetic chemicals.

This is the basis of the natural approach and will be discussed in more detail as we look at the various therapies that can be helpful to cystitis sufferers. Perhaps, ultimately, recurrent cystitis prob-lems will be solved once and for all, when barriers between 'orthodox' and 'alternative' are finally broken down and the two sides join forces for the benefit of their patients.

In the meantime, here is the approach you can expect a caring GP to follow, in treating your cystitis.

Case history
Let's pretend that you are visiting your GP because you have been

experiencing pain on passing urine, getting up once or twice at night to visit the bathroom, wanting to pass urine more frequently than usual during the day, and often passing only a few drops at a time.

Your doctor would want to know how long the symptoms had bothered you, and whether you had had them before. He would want to know about any accompanying symptoms (fever, loin pain), and whether your urine appeared darker than normal, pink or red in colour, or had an offensive smell.

He would also ask you – if you *had* had similar attacks in the past – when you had experienced the first attack, what tended to bring such attacks on, whether anything made them better or worse, whether you had been confined to bed with your symptoms and whether either of your parents, or other family members, tended to suffer similarly. (Tuberculosis is a rare contributory factor in certain cystitis cases; this would be relevant within a family, as might a tendency to form kidney or bladder stones, or to have an anatomical defect of the bladder or urethra.)

You would also very probably be questioned about your smoking habits. Further investigations at the hospital may entail a general anaesthetic, so the condition of your lungs is relevant. In addition, malignant tumours of the bladder and the kidneys are more likely to occur in smokers than in non-smokers.

Physical examination
This would include feeling your tummy, all over at first and then just above the pubic bone (where a full bladder can be felt), and around each kidney. A doctor examines a kidney manually by sliding his hand below the back of the patient lying supine on the examination couch, just behind the kidney area. He then explores deeply with his free, examining hand to reveal areas of tenderness, and/or any irregularity of the kidney's surface. Kidney swelling, or a kidney tumour, can often be felt in slim patients.

The doctor would listen to your chest, and probably take your blood-pressure. Again, both of these are relevant when a general anaesthetic is to be given in the near future, and certain disorders of the kidney can give rise to a raised blood-pressure. You would very likely be examined internally, too, if your urine had been blood-stained, or if you had symptoms suggestive of an inflamed vagina or cervix rather than, or as well as, an inflamed bladder and urethra.

After he had felt the inside of your vagina with an index finger, wearing a sterile glove lubricated with clear, odourless jelly, the doctor would insert a metal vaginal speculum (a slim 'duck's bill' shaped instrument which opens up inside you), enabling him to shine a light on to your cervix and inspect it for signs of infection and inflammation.

If, instead of this being your first visit, you were returning to the surgery with obstinately recurrent cystitis, your GP might also take swabs (smears of the cervix and vagina for bacteriological testing), obtained by wiping the appropriate area with a small pad of sterile cotton wool at the end of a slim wooden stick. You would be unlikely to feel anything while this was being done. An enthusiastic, or especially efficient, GP might go a step further, and take two swabs of your urethra, the first before massaging the urethra and the second following light massage of the area. ·

These swabs are important if your underlying problem is infection of the urethra without involvement of the bladder. The pre-massage swab would reveal bacterial infection inside the hollow of the urethra itself, and you may be asked for a separate urine specimen to indicate possible urethral bacteria, in which case only the first 5 millilitres (ml) of your urine stream would be required, rather than an MSU (see page 27).

The second (post-massage) swab would be taken in an attempt to show infection within the paraurethral glands, small mucus-secreting glands situated on either side of the urethra and opening into it by small ducts. These glands can be the site of infection, cyst formation or stone deposits, and if those at the upper end of the urethra are involved, stricture of this portion of the urethra may result with consequent obstruction to the passage of urine from the bladder.

Problems within the paraurethral glands, especially infection, would irritate the lining membrane and produce many of the symptoms of classic cystitis.

Some women refuse to visit their doctors if there is the slightest chance that an 'internal' will be performed. If you hate the idea, or it hurts, either tell your doctor and ask him to use plenty of KY lubricating jelly as you are nervous, or try to see a woman doctor. Internal examinations are, in fact, quick and painless, and there is no need whatever to feel embarrassed or frightened by them.

Urine specimen

A specimen of your urine is bound to be required. You can produce one in the toilets at the surgery, or take one with you to save time. If you do this, make sure that you use a *very clean* screwtop jar, with a lid that fits perfectly tightly. Whatever it has had in it before you use it for a specimen, do scrub it out with hot water and detergent and rinse it with plenty of fresh, clean water afterwards. Bacteria present from the jar's previous contents are likely to prove tenacious, and you are trying to produce a container to equal those with which your doctor's surgery is equipped, which are designed for the purpose and are sealed and sterile until opened.

Wherever you produce the specimen, choose if you can to do so when you have not taken any liquid for a few hours. Very dilute urine can appear to contain far fewer bacteria than concentrated urine, and if there are some present, you want to give them every chance to show themselves!

This is how to take a specimen. Before you start, it is worth filling in the details on the label of the jar, if you are using one from the doctor's surgery. A few drops of moisture on the label afterwards, makes this task very difficult. If you are using a home-improvized container, stick on a label with your name on it, the nature of the specimen (MSU), the name of your doctor, and the time the specimen was collected.

The urine specimen is known as an 'MSU' (mid-stream specimen of urine), and the object is to collect a sample (2-4 fl oz will do) mid-stream – i.e. after passing some, but not all, of the urine in your bladder. In this way, bacteria within the external opening of the urethra and on adjacent tissues, are washed away before the actual sample is collected.

Wash and dry your genital area. Pass a little urine into the lavatory and then stop the flow. Hold the specimen jar in position and pass a little urine into it. Remove the jar and screw on the lid, and finish opening your bladder as usual.

This is what happens to it in the hospital laboratory.

Bacteriological tests

The form accompanying the sample will have been filled in by your doctor. The request is usually made for 'microscopy, culture and sensitivity', so the first action taken is the viewing of a drop of the urine on a glass slide by means of a microscope. The pathologist, or one of his trained technicians, examines the slide for the presence of bacteria, blood cells and pus cells.

This can be done either by using the sample of urine as it is, and applying a biological stain to show up the bacteria, or by 'spinning the sample down' in an electric centrifuge in order to separate the solid matter in the urine from the liquid part. The sediment can then be placed under the microscope and scanned for bacteria, red and white blood cells, with or without the help of a staining technique.

'Culture' refers to applying drops of urine to a specially prepared culture plate, containing a thin layer of jellied broth. The broth resembles aspic jelly, and contains those nutrients most likely to encourage bacteria to grow and multiply. The urine drops are extended over the surface of the jelly by means of a metal spreader, and the lid replaced. The plate is then incubated overnight at the optimal temperature favouring bacterial growth, and the bacterial cultures, or colonies, that grow from infected urine, viewed the next morning.

These resemble small spots of mould similar to those seen on jam or jelly that has been left uncovered for several days. They are usually white or cream in colour, and some produce visible changes in the jelly broth around them. Others give off an offensive smell, and most common ones are sufficiently characteristic of their type to be easily recognized by the naked eye.

The sensitivity test shows the bacteria's reaction to a range of antibiotics. A sensitivity disc made of paper in the shape of a wheel with spokes, is impregnated with small amounts of the antibiotics commonly useful in the treatment of urinary tract infection. Examples include co-trimoxazole – Septrin; nalidixic acid with sodium citrate and bicarbonate – Mictral; the penicillin ampicillin – Penbritin. Each spoke end carries a different antibiotic, and the disc is placed flat on the surface of the culture medium plate.

The antibiotics to which the bacteria are sensitive (i.e. by which they are inhibited), are indicated by clear rings around those spokes, where the bacterial colonies have been unable to flourish. The report is then sent back to your doctor, naming the type of bacteria found in your urine specimen and the antibiotics most likely to succeed in getting rid of it.

What I have described above is the standard laboratory technique for the examination of a urine sample from a patient complaining of cystitis symptoms. Like all tests, however, it is subject to error, and it is possible to obtain both 'false positives' and 'false negatives'. What pathologists call 'bacteriuria' is, quite literally, the presence of bacteria in the urine. A falsely positive result may come about due to bacterial contaminants in the collection vessel, on the tissues around the urethral opening, in the urethra itself, or from gross contamination from vaginal secretions or from the faeces (motions).

A 'false negative' may be obtained if, for some reason, the bacteria are not seen on microscopy, and fail to flourish on the culture medium plate.

A degree of contamination is very common in a urine sample. The term 'significant bacteriuria' is used to denote the presence of 100,000 or more bacteria per ml of urine, a criterion accepted as a reliable definition of genuinely infected urine when the mid-stream specimen method is used correctly.

Further investigation

Your GP may suggest carrying out further investigations into your cystitis symptoms, if they persist despite several urine samples producing consistently negative results, or if you continue to suffer from bacterial cystitis attacks despite antibiotic treatment. He is almost bound to suggest a hospital appointment if blood has been present in your urine specimen.

These investigations are performed in a hospital, and their aim is to reveal any predisposing causes for the disorder (see page 24). Few people actually enjoy keeping hospital appointments and going for tests, so it is cheering to realize that these are far less likely to apply to you now you are aware of the dozens of different, non-infective causes of bladder and urethral infection.

All the same, it is reassuring to know that accurate, painless tests are available should you need to have them. They are unlikely to necessitate your spending more than twenty-four hours in the hospital, and, briefly, are likely to consist of the following:

Blood test
A sample of your blood will be taken for a full blood count, and to determine what is known as your 'biochemical profile'. The first of these reveals whether or not you are anaemic (which is quite possible if you have been losing a little blood in your urine over a period of weeks), and identifies and counts the different cells present. An increase in the number of white blood cells, for example, indicates that an infective cause of your cystitis symptoms is likely.

The 'biochemical profile' is done to rule out the possibility of kidney malfunction, and of secondary tumour deposits in liver and bones. The test would also reveal the likelihood of a prostate gland tumour in a male patient with cystitis symptoms and blood in his water.

These tests are standard procedures. Having a few millilitres of blood withdrawn from an arm vein is not painful, and the tests do not imply that the doctor suspects the presence of cancer or of any other disease he has not discussed with you.

MSU
You will be asked to provide a fresh mid-stream urine specimen. If there is any blood present, a count will be made of both the red and white blood cells, and cells denoting the presence of a tumour will also be looked for. The specimen will be tested for protein as well as for blood, and for 'casts', tiny fragments bearing the shape of the kidney tubules in which they are formed, and indicative of kidney disease.

The acidity will also be tested, and any pus cells noted. An acid urine with pus cells and no bacterial growth indicates a specific infection with organisms known as mycobacteria.

Endoscopy
For this investigation, you may either be given a general anaesthetic, or be allowed to remain conscious, while the surgeon passes the cystoscope viewing instrument into your bladder with

the help of jelly containing a local anaesthetic. Its object is to allow the lining of the bladder to be viewed (this is 'cystoscopy'), and the lining of the urethra as well ('urethroscopy'). For a long time, it was usual practice to examine the urethra in men only, but use cystoscopy for both men and women. Since the urethra is so much longer in the male, far more attention was paid to it. This is now realized to be a mistake, since a high proportion of the women suffering from 'recurrent cystitis' do not have inflamed bladders at all, but highly inflamed urethras.[2]

Both urethroscopy and cystoscopy give the surgeon the chance to check these areas for inflammation, small growths, bladder stones, or blind pouches that may harbour multiplying bacteria.

In the operating theatre, your feet would be raised in the air and suspended from stirrups (as they often are when a baby is delivered), and the surgeon would be seated on a stool at the foot of the operating table. A tube would be inserted into your bladder and any residual urine drained away. Sterile water would then be passed into your bladder via the tube, and the illuminated cystoscope viewing lens attached.

After examining the bladder lining, the cystoscope would either be withdrawn, or the surgeon would proceed to a further investigation, this time involving the two urine tubes (ureters).

It is now possible to examine the ureters visually, using a 'ureteroscope'. This is introduced through the urethra and bladder into each ureter where it enters the bladder, and passed up its length as far as the hollow ('pelvis') of the kidney. This permits small tissue samples (called 'biopsies') to be taken, should any of the viewed parts show signs of disease, and ureteric or kidney stones to be removed.

Ureteric catheterization
The object of this procedure is to introduce a catheter (fine tube) into each of the ureters in turn, and to obtain a urine sample from each of the kidneys. The end of the catheter may be introduced right up into the pelvis of the kidney, or only into the inside of the ureter.

This is done when a kidney infection is suspected as the cause of cystitis and urethritis symptoms. This possibility may be suspected on the grounds of the case history, since loin pain and fever generally indicate an infection higher up the urinary tract than the bladder, although their absence does not mean that kidney infection can be ruled out.

The urine samples are collected and placed in sterile containers clearly marked 'left' and 'right' (and woe betide the nurse, student or house surgeon who neglects to mark them and then confuses the two!).

The samples are examined as described above for an ordinary urine sample, except that the criterion of 100,000 bacteria per ml urine does not apply. Catheterization of the ureters or kidney pelvices is an aseptic technique, and, providing the specimen is not contaminated by incorrect handling prior to culture, any number of bacteria found in the specimen are regarded as signifying the presence of infection.

Intravenous urogram
This test is mandatory if your urine has contained blood. Also known as an intravenous pyelogram (or IVP), it is carried out in the X-ray department and is used to show the outline on an X-ray film or screen of your kidneys, ureters and bladder. This is achieved by injecting you with 'contrast medium', a substance which is concentrated and excreted by the kidneys and which shows up the outline of the urinary organs during the excretory process.

The contrast medium is a blue liquid which is injected slowly into a convenient arm vein. The process is painless and unalarming, but the radiographer should remember to mention that, as the dye enters your system, you may experience a 'pins and needles' sensation in your muscles, especially those of the upper and lower arm, and calf muscles.

If a micturating cystogram has also been requested, then you will be secured comfortably to the X-ray table, which will then be tilted until you are vertical. You will be supplied with a small dish, and asked to open your bladder into it, while the radiographer watches his X-ray screen to note whether the ureters fill the bladder normally. He will also be anxious to check whether, in turn, the urine passes in the expected way, down out of the bladder through the urethra, without encountering any obstacles, or showing any signs of thickened walls, kinks or abnormal urethral bulges.

Should anything abnormal be apparent from the X-ray films, then a further radiological test would be performed while you were in the operating theatre, to reveal further details of the disorder.

The theatre test is known as an ascending ureterogram. Radio opaque dye is passed into the bladder and up the ureters until the whole tract from the bladder up to the kidneys is visible on the screen of the TV monitor used for the purpose.

Any distortion of the collecting system by an abnormal mass (tumour) in either kidney, would be followed by a diagnostic ultrasound examination, which permits solid or cystic tumours larger than 1.5 cm (two-thirds of an inch) in diameter to be identified.

One of the most recently introduced diagnostic techniques is computerized axial tomography (CT scan). This is used for the investigation of kidney tumours, and is capable of detecting extremely small kidney growths. By choosing the right contrast media (radio-opaque dyes), it is also possible to pick up filling defects in the urinary collecting system of the kidneys and upper part of the ureters, as well as signs of tumour in the lower ureters and the bladder.

You may also have heard of 'NMR' (nuclear magnetic resonance) imaging. This is useful in the pelvic region, particularly in showing up tumours of the prostate, and tumours of the bladder prior to endoscopy.

Surgery may be indicated to remove any abnormal structures noted during the course of the previous exploratory techniques. Examples are the removal of a cystocoele or tumour within the bladder, a stone blocking either ureter or causing irritation within the bladder, or, rarely, the removal of a diseased kidney. In some women, an abnormally shaped urethra appears to be the explanation of the curative effect in a number of these cases, probably because the passage of the cystoscope up the urethra and into the bladder dilates the urethra and overcomes its tendency to 'kink'.

Some women suffer both from cystitis symptoms, and from difficulty in emptying their bladders completely. This is most commonly found in middle age, and one of the contributory causes can be weak action of the 'detrusor' muscle in the bladder wall, responsible for emptying the bladder by contracting and squeezing its contents. Slight prolapse of the bladder aggravates the situation, and this is worsened by the need to strain in order to pass urine, with consequent kinking or distortion of the urethra.

The bladder also tends to retain urine (which becomes stagnant and inflames the bladder lining) in women suffering from constipation, fibroids in the womb (uterus), or ovarian cysts. These are believed to affect the bladder by compressing the organs within the pelvis and distorting the normal shape of the urethra. Sometimes, a degree of obstruction to the passage of urine down the urethra occurs following the menopause. One of the changes occurring as a result of the fall in the blood level of oestrogen, is degeneration in the lining membrane of the urethra. Besides causing irritation and the frequent desire to pass water, the membrane changes can produce a relatively rigid and inelastic urethral tube, often associated with weak detrusor muscular action.

In the next chapter we will see how GPs and urological experts treat patients with confirmed bacterial cystitis, before going on to look at the approaches adopted by practitioners of several of the available alternative forms of treatment.

3

Orthodox Methods of Treatment

We saw in the last chapter the many different possible sources of urinary tract infection, all of which are capable of causing the symptoms of cystitis. I have given details of these problems, and of the diagnostic methods used in detecting them, because any woman with a burning pain on passing urine, combined with the need to visit the toilet frequently and the passage of dark, possibly blood-stained urine, *may* have any of the underlying disorders I have mentioned.

These problems can only be diagnosed satisfactorily in a hospital with the use of up-to-date technology and the interpretive skill of expert urologists and their staff. Should your doctor suggest hospital investigations to you, it is natural that you should want to know something about them, their purpose and how they are carried out. Doctors do not always have the time (or, regrettably, the willingness) to explain forthcoming tests to their patients. So details of possible ones have been included in this book to allay any apprehensions you may feel about a forthcoming hospital appointment.

Do bear in mind, though, that common disorders have common causes. Infections of the urinary tract are the second most common infection to be seen by general practitioners (the most common of all being infections of the ear, nose and throat – upper respiratory tract). Very few cases of cystitis turn out to be due to tumours, and not many – considering the number of cases seen yearly – turn out to be due to a stone in the kidney or ureter, or to structural abnormalities. So please do not assume that you have something appalling wrong with you, just because your symptoms are going to be investigated at the hospital. If your urine is infected, misuse of toilet paper (see page 17) or urethral contamination during love-making, are many times more likely causes.

Doctors who have specialized in urological medicine are, without doubt, the best people to treat complex kidney and bladder problems, when malignant tumours, infection or anatomical defects are apparent. All the same, as I mentioned earlier, there is every reason in favour of your turning to alternative methods of treatment as an adjunct to the orthodox therapy necessary on such occasions. Most specialists – and GPs for that matter – would wish you to consult them, if you decided to bolster their attempts to cure you with, say, homoeopathic remedies, acupuncture or hypnotherapy for relaxation. Most people would probably do so, anyway, out of courtesy, although a lot would depend upon the relationship that existed between them and their consultant or family doctor.

Very few doctors, however, would be likely to object, and some of the more progressive ones may well suggest a suitable alternative themselves, to be used in combination with the treatment scheme they had devised.

Getting orthodox treatment for some of the possible causes of cystitis, however, still leaves a tremendous amount of room for self-help and self-management methods. Only around 50 per cent (or less) of cases of cystitis turn out to be due to infection, and the most sensible approach is to know when to visit your doctor (or call him in!), and when to manage the attack without his help, either alone or with the assistance of an alternative therapist.

Having made these points, I will give a brief account of orthodox treatment and the reasons why certain standard measures are adopted. Fewer people (especially cystitis patients) would pay unnecessary visits to their doctor, if they understood what he (in the name of modern medicine) is able to do, and what is quite beyond him. Conversely, more people who really do need help and are either too shy or too frightened to ask for it (fears of that 'internal' again?), might well pluck up courage and ring for an appointment at the surgery if they knew how very unfrightening a simple physical examination is. Here, then, is the course of action your doctor will be likely to take when he has had a positive report back from the hospital showing that your urine was infected.

The report

The type of bacterial organisms detected by the bacteriological tests is significant. The most likely variety is E. coli, and the next most likely is Proteus mirabilis. Others quite commonly found include Staphylococcus albus, and Micrococcus. These names may not mean much to you. But your doctor might mention the findings, including the sort of bacteria found, and the importance of the above four types is that they are all suggestive of uncomplicated infection in a normally functioning urinary tract.

Other varieties of bacteria which may be identified include the Klebsiella species, the Enterobacter species and the Proteus species (other than the 'mirabilis' variety); Streptococcus faecalis; and Psuedomonas aeruginosa. The presence of these bacteria, especially in recurrent urinary infections, may indicate an abnormality of the urinary tract. Your doctor would be likely to suggest some hospital investigations to check the underlying cause of the problem.

Choice of antibiotic

His choice of treatment would be guided by the sensitivity findings on the laboratory report. If the bacterial type and/or its sensitivity were not known, then treatment selection would be guided by his knowledge of the common resistance patterns in the district. That is to say that, while it is well known that bacteria succeed in altering their structure from time to time, in such a way that a particular strain grows resistant to a variety of antibiotic drug to which it was hitherto susceptible (sensitive), not everybody realizes that the resistances put up against a particular antibiotic can differ from district to district.

A bacterial type that may succumb easily to ampicillin (Penbritin), for example, in Cornwall, may have developed a fair degree of resistance to it in Staffordshire! When this is the case, another antibiotic to which that bacterial strain is likely to be sensitive is chosen instead. Personal knowledge of local bacterial sensitivities is, for that reason, a very valuable part of successful treatment.

Method of treatment

Uncomplicated urinary infection in young women is generally

treated with a short course of antibiotics, either as a single high dose or for one to three days. Likely antibiotics in this instance include nalidixic acid (Mictral), amoxycillin (Amoxil), or a sulphonamide (e.g. Kelfizine). Recurrent infection in women (and all infections in men) should be treated with a full course of antibiotics using conventional dosage. Likely antibiotic choices for this type of treatment include co-trimoxazole (Septrin, Chemotrim), ampicillin (Penbritin) and trimethoprim (Monotrim).

If the infection is related to predisposing factors, then the treatment should be tailored to the needs of the individual patient and may be needed for many months. (It is in this kind of situation that supplementary treatment from an alternative therapist would prove especially useful, if aimed at boosting the patient's immune defence system and helping her to overcome infection successfully.)

All antibiotic drugs prescribed for urinary infections are present in high concentrations in the urine, and it is not necessary for the doctor to take the patient's physical size into consideration when deciding upon dosage, as he may well do when, for instance, treating a chest infection. Thus, whether you weigh a hefty 17 st (108 kg), or a slim, slight 8 st (51 kg), your dosage will be identical. If, however, there are any indications of kidney infection (as mentioned above, these are likely to be loin pain and fever), the concentration of the drug in the blood-stream is very significant and this would mean that the dosage should be adjusted according to body weight.

Alternatively, the antibiotic of choice might be administered as an intramuscular injection, rather than by mouth, in order to increase the speed with which it was absorbed into the blood-stream. (High doses of antibiotic, often in injection form, are needed to treat male patients with an infected prostate gland problem, since most drugs enter the tissue of this gland slowly and inadequately.)

A wide variety of oral drugs are available for the treatment of urinary tract infection, but where the bacteria concerned are sensitive to the antibiotic chosen, the cure rates are much the same (between 85 and 90 per cent). Most strains of E. coli have retained their sensitivity to sulphonamides (e.g. Gantrisin, Kelfizine, Urolucosil), and consequently these are often the first choice of therapy. Co-trimoxazole or trimethoprim provide alternatives to the sulphonamides, but more bacterial strains are developing resistance to these drugs.

Nitrofurantoin (Furadantin, Macrodantin, Berkfurin) is familiar to many cysistis sufferers. It has to be taken together with food or a drink; but it has a good record in dealing effectively with post-coital (after love-making) cystitis, and it is useful when a long-term, low-dose form of treatment is indicated. For patients with a hypersensitivity to penicillin, nalidixic acid (Mictral, Negram, Uriben) can be a valuable alternative.

Follow-up of treatment

I am mentioning the necessity for follow-up treatment after a course of antibiotics for urinary tract infection, in case either your GP forgets to ask you to return to have your urine checked, or you assume that to make a further appointment is a waste of your GP's time and your own, since you are symptom-free.

Although your doctor may not have sent off a sample of your urine before starting you on a course of antibiotics, nevertheless your urine must be shown to be free from infection once the treatment is over. If the cystitis attack is your first, or one of a very few over a long period of time, then a specimen needs to be checked only once, seven to ten days after you have finished the antibiotic course.

If, however, you suffer from the menace of recurrent attacks, a further specimen sent one month later may prove useful. Where men are concerned, both one-week and four-week checks are essential, since even a simple infection may be associated with bacterial infection of the prostate gland, and this may cause recurrent infections.

If you are given a long-term course of antibiotics, then you should have your urine tested as a matter of routine, every four to eight weeks. At the same time, you should have a full blood count done and possibly biochemical blood tests as well, to check for any sign of the possible long-term side-effects of the antibiotic you are receiving.

One of the most important things you can know about recurrent cystitis attacks which show bacterial infection, especially if your attacks are associated with fever and loin pain (pain below the ribs at the back, over the two kidney areas), is that you MUST have an IVP (see 'Intravenous Urogram' in Chapter 2) to discover whether your kidneys are possibly the source of the problem.

Side-effects

All of the various antibiotics so far mentioned, can cause their own particular range of side-effects. There is insufficient space available to look at them all, so I will briefly mention the adverse side-effects of two of them – Septrin and Penbritin.

Septrin

This can cause nausea, vomiting, inflammation of the tongue, diarrhoea and skin rashes. Colitis can result on rare occasions, as can severe skin sensitivity reactions. Septrin's sulphonamide content can also produce changes in the blood, including a shortage of blood platelets – which affects clotting of the blood – and a shortage of some of the white cells. Most of these have been found to be reversible on withdrawal from the drug.

Subjective (non-scientifically testable) complaints have included headache, depression, dizziness and hallucinations, but their relationship to the drug is unproven.

During long-term therapy, changes in the bone marrow have occurred in isolated cases. These are in no way associated with malignant changes in the bone marrow such as those associated with leukaemia, and they are reversible by doses of folinic acid.

Penbritin

Nausea, vomiting, headaches and slight dizziness can result from the use of penicillin. It can cause diarrhoea, and skin rashes are a common side-effect. The main types of rash have been described. One is similar to 'hives' or 'nettle rash', and appears as large, itchy, white blobs surrounded by inflamed skin. This is probably a true urticarial rash and indicative of genuine penicillin hypersensitivity.

The other rash type is a bright red one typical of ampicillin (a non-proprietary name for penicillin). It is especially likely to occur in patients suffering from glandular fever (infectious mononucleosis) and is an indication for stopping the treatment.

It is also well worth mentioning the other common outcome of antibiotic therapy – monilia, or 'thrush' infection. This results from the effect of the antibiotics on the useful bacteria normally resident within the bowel, which are able to keep the growth of harmful organisms within the intestine under control.

Weakening the strength of the protective organisms allows the 'thrush' yeast organism to thrive, and outbreaks of it frequently appear both within the intestine and, in women, inside the vagina. Some recurrent cystitis (or urethritis) sufferers are unlucky enough to have an attack of 'thrush' vaginitis following every antibiotic course they are obliged to take to get rid of their urinary infections.

It is little wonder that, after a few attacks of each, they find it difficult to tell whether they are currently suffering from a burning within the urethra (and bladder), or whether they have a sore vagina due to the scalding of the inflamed labia that occurs each time they open their bladders.

Oestrogen therapy

We have seen that the urethra lies in front of the vagina, in close proximity to it. It is, in fact, actually embedded in the front wall of the vagina (although, of course, the two passageways are completely discrete from one another), and the lower part of the urethra actually develops from the same embryonic duct as the vagina, while the baby is in the womb.

Because of this, the effects of a declining oestrogen level upon the lining of the vagina (producing degeneration, dryness and soreness) are frequently shared by the urethra. This is one of the causes for the urinary symptoms that show themselves during or after the menopause, e.g. 'frequency' (having to spend a penny more often than usual), irritation within the urethra, and having to get up at night to pass water.

Sometimes, patients with this variety of urethritis show persistent urinary symptoms with pus in the urine but no signs of bacterial infection. It is particularly common in the elderly post-menopausal woman, and many doctors prescribe a three-month course of hormone replacement therapy (HRT – oestrogen in combination with progestogen) to clear up the problem.

The lower end of the urethra can actually be lost, due to oestrogen deficiency. If oestrogen is given early enough, consultant urological surgeon Mr Patrick Smith was reported in *GP*, the weekly newspaper for GPs, as saying, 'these changes can be aborted and the urethra restored'.

If not, they [the patients] may go on to develop urethral stricture from chronic inflammatory scarring and dilatation of the upper tract [because of the back pressure due to the obstruction further down].

What might be mistaken for a urethral polyp in such women could well be prolapse of the upper urethra as a result of lower urethral tissue loss. The problem can be quickly righted by three months' hormonal replacement therapy. (*GP*, 17 May 1985.)

Surgery

We have already seen that anatomical abnormalities can account for persistent infection in the urinary system, and that these, as well as renal and ureteric stones, can be treated readily with modern surgery. We have also seen that cystoscopy can have a 'magically' curative effect in a number of women with recurrent urethral and bladder symptoms, possibly by correcting an oddly shaped urethra and bladder neck dysfunction.

There is a further instance in which your doctor might recommend that you see a urological surgeon, who may, in turn, suggest a minor operation to you. That is, if you suffer from recurrent bouts of the 'urethral syndrome', are still of reproductive age and are not helped very much by antibiotics. It has been found that many women with these factors in common, have their urethras tethered inside their vaginas by remnants of the hymen.

A short 'day case' surgical manoeuvre rectifies this problem. A further operation that has helped some of these women is removal of a small segment of the lower end of the urethra.

Symptomatic treatment

As we will see when we take a look at alternative approaches to the problem of cystitis, alternative practitioners regard the prescribing of antibiotics as 'symptomatic treatment', i.e. aimed only at the relief of a symptom, and failing to get to the root cause of the matter. This is because they see susceptibility to infections as a weakness needing correction; they regard the bacteria simply as a trigger factor that has sparked off overt symptoms and signs of inner imbalance.

Orthodox doctors, however, feel that in prescribing antibiotics, they *are* attacking the problem at its basic point, and are not, by and large, willing to believe that their method of treatment is in any way lacking. Since we, at medical school, are taught that bacteria, viruses and fungi *are* the causes of infections, and from the orthodox viewpoint this can easily be substantiated, few of us are prepared to look further than a positive bacteriological report for the 'cause' of a patient's cystitis.

This is especially the case when no predisposing factors such as anatomical anomalies can be found to explain the presence of the infection, and it does indeed give the appearance of having come 'out of the blue' through the medium of invading bacteria.

So to clear up what I mean in this book by 'symptomatic treatment', I am using the term as orthodox doctors would understand it since this chapter is dealing exclusively with orthodox methods of treatment. Killing the bacteria with antibiotic compounds is directed to the 'cause' either of proven bacterial cystitis, or what may turn out to be bacterial cystitis (since, nowadays, few doctors wait for the laboratory report on a urine specimen to be returned with a positive result before starting their patients on antibiotic therapy – see pages 16 and 17).

Besides antibiotic therapy, your doctor is also likely to advise you to rest in bed until the attack has subsided – that is, if you are not already there, and incapable of getting up and looking after yourself anyway!

Cystitis attacks differ a great deal, from one individual to another, in their severity, and while some sufferers 'soldier on', and continue to go to work, look after their families and go about life as normal, others feel too ill to put on a brave face. This is by far the most sensible reaction, and not only should you go to bed when you can feel an attack starting, but continue to rest until the symptoms have disappeared.

As well as *bed rest*, your GP would probably advise you to drink as much as possible. He may not say what you should drink, what you ought to avoid drinking, how much you should try to swallow, and over what period of time. Apart from saying that water is the best drink during a cystitis attack, and to warn you away from alcohol and tea and coffee, we will postpone details of your *liquid intake* until the final chapter, which is devoted to the subject of 'self-help' measures.

You may also be handed a prescription for that old-fashioned horror, 'Mist. Pot. Cit' (potassium citrate mixture). The instruction on the bottle of greenish liquid you received from your chemist would tell you to measure out 10 ml and drink it in a tumbler of water three times daily. Unfortunately, the taste is unbelievably repulsive; but if you were to take it, you would probably be pleasantly surprised.

Like many old-fashioned remedies, it works very well, and relieves the burning pain of cystitis and urethritis by alkalizing the urine. This means an end to the irritation of red, sore lining membrane by constant contact with acid.

Alternatively, you might be prescribed Pyridium (phenazo-pyridine hydrochloride), taken in tablet form, in a dose of two tablets three times daily after food. This is a urinary analgesic (pain killer), and can be taken with antibiotics if they are also prescribed. Your urine will be orange to red in colour while you are taking Pyridium, but it reverts to normal once you stop the tablets. If any of the coloured urine gets on to clothing, it should be washed out as soon as possible in warm, soapy water. The stain may be permanent.

An alternative to Pyridium is Urispas (flavoxate hydrochloride), also taken in tablet form, two, three times daily (relation to food unspecified). Urispas is an antispasmodic, selective to the muscle fibres throughout the urinary system, which it relaxes and makes pain-free. Urispas can be taken together with antibiotic therapy.

You may also be prescribed Urispas in hospital, where it is sometimes used before cystoscopy, and after any surgical inter-vention within the bladder or urethra when muscle spasm results from the unusual stimulation. It is unsuitable for anyone suffering from potentially obstructive conditions such as duodenal or pyloric obstruction, gastrointestinal haemorrhage, intestinal tumours and obstructive conditions of the bladder or urethra.

In the next chapter, we will see what the alternative therapies have to offer the cystitis sufferer, starting with naturopathy; and establish what is meant by the underlying principle of 'holism'.

4

An Alternative Approach

The principle of holism is fundamental to all the main varieties of alternative therapy. It is based on the concept of Man as a 'whole' being, consisting of body, mind and spirit, all three parts being of equal importance, and all being interdependent. All forms of holistic treatment take Man's three-sided nature into account, and never aim solely at curing, for instance, a bodily disorder without considering both the illness (and the treatment) in relation to the patient mentally and spiritually.

The concept of 'life force', or 'vital energy' is of great importance to holistic therapies. Difficult to define in precise terms, the 'life force' is that element which is present during the life of a plant, animal or human being, and so clearly absent once death has occured. It would be easy, and tempting, to wax poetical on the subject of the life force (the Chinese call it 'Ch'i'), and eulogize over its manifestation in all living things in the natural world.

Examples of its presence are legion, and apparent to all who look around them. A few instances which leap to mind are – a germinating seed on your windowsill, a puppy playing in the sunlight, birds flying cloudwards, two happy people running across a meadow, holding hands and laughing.

Everything that lives has a share of the life force, and all dead, decaying things lack it. And while there has been an enormous amount of dispute about the life force's actual nature, evidence has mounted over the past two decades demonstrating its existence in a number of different forms.

Evidence for the life force

Energy pathways are now known to exist along the *acupuncture meridians* recognized for thousands of years by the Chinese. Much has been written about them in orthodox medical literature, and research scientists are now convinced of their reality. A detailed article about acupuncture appearing in *GP* in 1984,[3] summed up the testable qualities both of meridian lines and of acupuncture points, and emphasized that 'acupuncture should be fully integrated within conventional medicine' (acupuncture is dealt with in further detail in Chapter 8).

Life force has been further demonstrated by the phenomenon of *Kirlian photography*. This technique was believed to have been discovered in the fifties by accident, when a Russian electronic technician, Semyon Kirlian, was called to mend some instruments at a research institute.[4] He saw a patient receiving electrotherapy, and noticed small light flashes between the electrodes and the patient's skin. Kirlian discovered that he could produce a picture of the electrical interaction by placing a photographic plate between skin and electrode.

It is now thought that the phenomenon was first observed and demonstrated by a Russian engineer Kakov Narkevich-Todko, in 1898.

Basic energy imbalances can be detected by this technique, which employs an electric camera emitting high-voltage, high-frequency, low-amperage impulses consisting of a combination of photons and cold electron emission. The high-frequency electro-magnetic field thus produced, interacts with the energy field surrounding living things to produce light, and create images which can be captured on photographic paper.

It is possible to photograph a person's entire energy field by these means, but it is more convenient to take pictures of the energy stream emitted from the fingers and the toes. Some aspects of the significance and interpretation of Kirlian photography are still controversial, but 'there is good correlation with basic energy levels'.[5] Because many meridians start or finish on the fingers and toes, Kirlian photography can be used to diagnose dysfunction at the meridian level, and can be employed usefully in combination with acupuncture as a pre- and post-treatment visual check.

The electromagnetic field of which we now have evidence

(whose source is the 'vital energy' within), has been equated with the *aura*. The word 'aura' has long been associated in many people's minds with the paranormal, and people who claim to be able to see it have been considered by many to be either exceptionally psychic, or persistently fraudulent, or subject to hallucinations.

Kirlian photographic images are, therefore, representations of the aura. No one has yet explained how some gifted individuals are able to see the aura of living things around them, while the rest of us cannot. However, this is a gift shared by many sane, rational and highly intelligent people who have no motivation to fraudulence and indeed often possess powers of healing that they use to the benefit of others. My own suggestion is that possessing this faculty is rather like possessing psychic 'double joints'!

People with physical 'double joints' (which are not really double, but which have a far greater range of mobility than normal due to the structure of surrounding muscles and ligaments), can contort their limb joints into the most astonishing configurations because they happen to be born with that particular knack. The same, I believe, applies to psychic faculties, and to certain intellectual ones. Examples are the innate possession of a superhuman memory for rows of ten or twenty digit figures, for instance, or the ability to recall pages of numbers from a table of logarithms.

None of these gifts is 'occult', weird or frightening. Just unusual. The normal aura is a clear blue, of even shape, and with no breaks in it, or signs of asymmetry. It changes colour, however, when the individual is ill, under stress, or taking drugs; and is disturbed when alcohol has been consumed. The department of medical photography at the Charing Cross hospital, London, has carried out experiments aimed at standardizing the Kirlian technique, to test its efficacy as a diagnostic tool.

The researchers discovered that carefully balanced and controlled conditions were necessary to obtain satisfactory aura pictures. The result, for instance, could be influenced by atmospheric conditions, temperature, humidity, and especially by the state of ionization of the air. Feelings of anger, depression or elation also influence the human aura; and alcohol was found to cause the subject's aura to grow spiky, change colour from blue to orange, and to fragment.

Orange was also found to creep into the aura when a subject had had a bad day. The main problem, said Mr Robin Williams, director of medical illustration at the Charing Cross hospital, was that all disturbed auras looked similar to one another, and it was impossible to tell from looking at a picture of one, whether the person was suffering from the effects of depression, physical illness or the effects of alcohol consumption.

Some researchers claim that cancer tissue has a distinct energy form which is demonstrable at a very early stage; but Mr Williams does not accept the truth of such statements. He does, however, acknowledge a relationship between the aura and acupuncture points. Kirlian photography maps out an energy field; and the pictures repeatedly showed little dots in the position of acupuncture points.

The following information, taken from an article by Doctor Maureen Swanson (GP, 5 October 1984) provides an example of the use of Kirlian photography in the indication of bodily malfunction. It illustrates the different picture which often occurs between the hands and feet of a patient. An approximate indication of energy levels can be determined by taking the electrical resistance across the upper and lower halves of the body. They are made by the patient holding an electrode in each hand, or standing on the electrode placed just behind the ball of each foot. High resistance readings indicate low energy. Individuals with no symptoms have hand-to-hand resistance measurements in the range 20 to $30\,\mathrm{k\Omega}$, and foot-to-foot readings of 30 to 40 $\mathrm{k\Omega}$.

Clinical experience over the last few years, however, has shown that a number of symptoms and illnesses can be classified depending upon whether or not an energy imbalance exists in the top or bottom half of the body. An excess of energy in the top half is found in the presence of allergies, headaches, migraine, nervous tension, asthma and insomnia.

Severe energy deficiencies across the bottom half of the body tend to indicate depressive illness and osteoarthritis.

Usually, the commonest energy imbalance seems to be an excess of energy across the top half of the body, and a lack of energy across the lower half. By stimulating specific acupuncture points, the energy levels can be manipulated. The resistance readings show how therapy is progressing from treatment session to treatment session. As readings approach the healthy level, symptoms abate.

In this way, for instance, a migraine sufferer can come for a check-up periodically, and if the resistance readings are starting to drift out of the normal range, one or two basic treatments can be given to restore them to their correct values, leaving the patient free of symptoms.

It is highly likely that the same approach could be adopted towards many other minor – and maybe not so minor – disorders, for example, recurrent attacks of cystitis and urethritis. The type of attacks that occur due to an abnormally sensitive bladder and urethral lining, is particularly likely to be associated with energy imbalance and therefore to be amenable to energy level correction.

The photograph that follows, reproduced by the kind permission of *GP*, illustrates the different picture I have just described as occurring frequently between hands and feet. High energy shown on the hand-to-hand conductance measurement shows as a faint image. This is because, in high energy states, light at the red end of

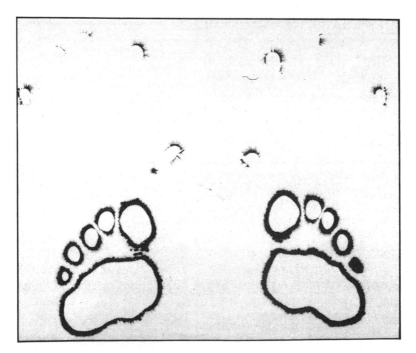

the spectrum is emitted which does not register on black and white photographic paper. This is termed a 'basic condition' because it affects the whole area of the hands. In this case, the patient was suffering from severe headaches which can be corrected using 'basic' acupuncture points.

The only 'system element' out of balance appears on the little toe of the right foot. A dark image can be seen, indicating degeneration due to emission at the violet end of the spectrum. The acupuncture meridians which start and finish on this toe are the kidney and bladder meridians. A one-sided imbalance, such as appears here, always results in severe symptoms of discomfort in the patient.

Tracing of the bladder meridian reveals that a 'point bladder 2' situated on the forehead is electrically abnormal. This point represents the frontal sinus. A suitable form of treatment would be auricular acupuncture on the sinus and bladder 'organ points', and a key point for the bladder meridian situated on the feet.

A recently developed technique, electrocrystal therapy, grew from discoveries made by Mr Harry Oldfield, a science graduate and schoolmaster who developed a great interest in the effects of Kirlian photography in the late seventies. He read about the 'phantom leaf' effect which, under very carefully controlled conditions, permits a photographic image to be made of the leaf of a plant showing the electromagnetic field of the entire leaf *despite the fact that seconds before, a fragment of it (up to 10 per cent) had been cut off*.

This phantom image shows that the life force of a plant lingers for a very brief time interval after part of its living structure has been removed, and it is interesting to note that this experiment will work (with a great deal of patience!) only when *organically grown* plants are used.

Mr Oldfield discovered that other ways existed besides Kirlian photography for exploring the nature of the life force and its electromagnetic field or aura. Analysing the energy field stimulated by Kirlian photographic methods, he found that it included electromagnetic energy at radio and audio frequencies as well as light. The original Kirlian apparatus used stimulating energy with a radio frequency of 2,000 kHz (identical with Radio 4 Long Wave). Other frequencies had been used in later experiments, resulting in different types of image. Mr Oldfield designed equipment to produce a source of stimulating energy from below the range of human hearing up through the audio range to radio frequency.

It operates from a 9-volt battery and the energy it produces can safely be used to merge with the body's own electromagnetic field to produce electromagnetic pulsation in the audio frequency range. An interesting revelation was that every individual's energy field responds to the stimulus of one basic frequency and its harmonics, the fundamental frequency varying from individual to individual. Mr Oldfield stresses that the effect is one of electromagnetic resonance, due to fluctuation in the energy field, not actual physical vibration of the body's tissues. It can be detected by a special probe, a sensitive sound level meter, or a nearby cassette tape recorder.

Mr Oldfield next developed a scanning method for detecting disturbances in the human energy field. The subject is given an insulated transducer to hold in one hand, while the therapist scans the stimulated energy field close to the subject's body with an electromagnetic probe. The generator is first tuned for peak response at the subject's natural resonance, by asking the subject to identify a healthy 'control' area on his or her body. The inner surface of an elbow is a common place for this purpose. Any area of the body which is out of energy balance, or harmony, with the whole person, responds less energetically to the induced frequency, in comparison with the optimal area. The natural frequency of a person with a debilitating disease affecting all their systems, such as disseminated cancer, can be difficult to detect.

The signal from the probe can be displayed on an oscilloscope together with the original signal from the generator, which enables disturbances to be seen easily. Experienced and intuitive users of this scanning technique are generally able to detect past and present weaknesses from the scan, and to foretell likely future ones. Many GPs have been impressed (if sometimes surprised) by the accuracy of the diagnoses made in this way.

The diagnostic scope of this technique soon led to its therapeutic application. Patients often reported relief from their symptoms after having a diagnostic scan. The name 'bio-entrainment' has been used in this context, meaning that the powerful electromagnetic signal 'reminds' the body's energy field of its normal and healthy state. Mr Oldfield began to investigate the effects of various frequencies and wave forms, and found that particular frequency bands could be used to stimulate and strengthen the energy field, others to balance it, and yet others to calm it down.

Crystals and gem stones entered the picture when Mr Oldfield tested their traditionally renowned healing powers with his measuring equipment and discovered that when they are stimulated by an electromagnetic field, a more powerful field results. In this way, it has been possible to combine the traditional healing properties of gem stones with the appropriate electromagnetic frequencies. Three gem stone groups have been found to enhance the special effects of stimulation (ruby, garnet etc.), balancing (jade, emerald etc.), and calming (sapphire, amethyst).

One interesting effect is that holding a crystal in the hand or wearing it as jewellery, produces an effect that can be picked up on an EEG (electro-encephalogram), a machine used by neurologists for examining people's brain waves (the electrical activity in the brain's cortex, or outer layer).

In many cases it is possible to relieve symptoms and to bring relief from pain. What actually happens at a treatment session, is that the diagnostic scan is first performed, the electromagnetic probe being in contact with a series of small crystals enclosed in a test-tube containing brine (which facilitates electrical conduction). Instead of covering the entire energy field around the body, the nuclei of concentrated energy (the chakras) situated at various levels along the length of the brain and spinal cord, are scanned. The spinal cord is the 'motorway' of (electrical) nervous impulses running between the brain and nerve supply to the rest of the body. The chakras, further mentioned in Chapter 9 dealing with relaxation techniques and yoga, clearly indicate where specific organs and body areas require further investigation and energy balancing.

After the diagnostic scan, the test-tube containing crystals of an appropriate type is applied to the affected area. A severe migraine has been terminated within ten minutes, and the acute pain of cystitis relieved in seven to eight minutes. The appropriate chakra or chakras are then treated, and a final scan taken to see the extent to which the energy readings have improved.

Holistic concept of health

A healthy person is one who possesses the life force in abundance, and has the physical, spiritual and mental aspects of his personal self in perfect balance. Disease is seen as the result of an unnatural lifestyle which hampers, instead of encouraging, the growth and development of Man's whole being.

An example of how our lifestyle can work against us is the high incidence of many diseases directly associated with Western civilization. Of particular note are heart attacks, strokes, arterial and venous (veins) disease, many forms of cancer (including bladder cancer), many mental disorders, and (although not in most cases ranking in gravity with the diseases so far mentioned) cystitis and urethritis.

These and many others – have been related directly to the type of food we eat (cancer, heart and circulatory disease, cystitis), our sedentary lifestyles (most disorders), our refusal to learn and practise relaxation, the smoking habits of many of us (this encourages bladder cancer as well as lung cancer), our abuse of drugs and alcohol, and the multitude of stresses to which we are continually subject for much of the time we are awake.

The alternative, or natural, therapies aim at correcting the imbalances they detect in our life force, by a variety of means. The acupuncturist, for instance, works by liberating blocked energy pathways (meridians) within the body by the insertion of needles at specific points.

The herbalist seeks to redress imbalance and to increase the flow of vital energy by utilizing the harmonizing properties of plants and herbs, chosen not only for their medicinal properties but also for their more esoteric qualities associated with age-old beliefs and experience.

The naturopath sets about correcting a patient's energy imbalance by stimulating the innate healing powers we all possess by natural means, and by helping him to correct those elements of his lifestyle that are most likely to be contributing to his disorder.

5

Naturopathic Treatment

Naturopathy
Naturopathy is a system of alternative medicine based upon the healing power of nature. It regards the human person (and every living organism) as essentially able to heal itself, given the right conditions. Those 'conditions' refer to lifestyle, environment and the number and nature of stress factors encountered by the individual, and it is these that the naturopath aims at reorganizing to meet the needs of each individual patient.

Theory
There is ample evidence that we possess self-healing powers. During an attack of bacterial cystitis, for instance, the lining of the bladder and urethra becomes inflamed, and as we saw in an earlier chapter, inflammation is one of the body's cardinal defence mechanisms. The inflammatory process is a deliberate attempt, frequently successful, to restore the body to a healthy state, through marshalling the body's forces against harmful stimuli.

The epithelial lining of the lower urinary tract becomes engorged with dilated capillaries, and the white blood cells leak outwards through their walls, and engulf and destroy E. coli bacteria that have ascended from the urethra. Small cracks in the urethral lining open up, causing intense pain as hot, acid urine washes over them. It can increase your distress a great deal when, in addition to the pain you are experiencing, you find traces of blood and pus in your water.

Yet the blood is a sign that the body's defence forces are winning important battles, and even while the blood oozes from the opened-up cracks in the urethral lining, the body's blood clotting mechanism is being brought into action, utilizing prothrombin and the tiny blood platelets to seal up the cracks.

The presence of a certain amount of pus is also a 'good' sign. It consists of cellular debris shed during the inflammatory process, white cells which have engulfed bacteria, and the dead bacteria themselves, and is evidence that your bladder lining is putting up a good fight against its invaders.

It may, nevertheless, be difficult for you to feel much appreciation for the inflammatory defence mechanism, when you are sitting in the loo at three in the morning, passing tiny drops of blood-stained urine that feel like glass spicules. And it would be asking too much to expect you to applaud nature's cleverness in designing this mechanism when there are no bacteria to be overcome, i.e. your lining membrane has been aroused to a state of heat and pain through urethral irritation due to scented talcum powder, vaginal deodorant or soap.

Your delicate urethral lining, however, cannot 'know' the difference between foreign bacterial invaders and synthetic chemicals. The latter may not be actually harmful, but they are noxious substances as far as the intimate lining of your urinary tract is concerned, and it reacts accordingly. The answer is to avoid bringing it into contact with whatever upsets it.

Other examples of self-healing are equally easy to find. Fractured bones mend; cuts heal; burns become covered with new skin or, at least, protective scar tissue; and torn muscle fibres undergo repair. All of these instances of self-correction, naturopaths attribute to the individual's 'life force' (the energy we have discussed in the last chapter). Another, less precise term for it, in this instance, might be 'vitality'.

Health

According to naturopathic theory, health is expressed in terms of the individual's capacity for withstanding disease, otherwise referred to as his 'capacity for function'. A person of full functional capacity would be extremely unlikely to fall prey to any kind of disease at all.

If you suffer from recurrent cystitis, for instance, and feel generally below par for most of the time, you are likely to continue to succumb to attacks. If you take measures to increase your 'illness-withstanding' powers, however, through a more nutritious diet, regular exercise and daily relaxation, then the intervals between attacks are likely to grow longer and longer until, given the right conditions, they disappear for good.

Symptoms of disease, on the other hand, are regarded as evidence of the body's fighting capacity against illness. Experiencing an acute attack of cystitis and regaining health afterwards, would be applauded as proof of inherent stamina, and stalwart defence mechanisms. The inflammatory process involved is regarded as a 'healing crisis', and a necessary part of the process of recovery. Feverish colds, catarrh, the occasional vomiting attack, even a bout of cystitis, are regarded by some naturopaths as serving a normalizing purpose, and a sign that the body's vital force is restoring equilibrium by cleansing itself of toxic waste.

This state of (dynamic) equilibrium which naturopaths equate with health depends upon the harmonious interfunction of three major factors: the structural, the biochemical and the emotional. A structurally healthy person is free from muscle tension, postural strain, malfunctioning joints and disturbed nerve conduction. Hence his circulatory system functions normally and his vital organs are both well-nourished and free from toxic accumulation.

Biochemical health results from adequate and appropriate nutrition, combined with the ability to utilize the products of digestion for the myriad bodily functions which require them.

Emotional and mental stability depends upon the integrity of the other two factors, and also contributes to their harmonious interaction.

Disease

Naturopaths regard disease as a disturbance in the body's natural equilibrium due to a disruptive influence that the body's homoeostatic mechanisms have been unable to overcome. 'Homoeostasis' refers to the innate 'self-righting' mechanism we have just described, which seeks to maintain inner stability and harmony between the three vital factors. The individual is believed to succumb to such a disruptive force, as a result of both prenatal and postnatal causal factors, which bring about a decline in cellular vitality (otherwise known as 'mesotrophy').

Prenatal causal factors predisposing the individual to ill health include inherited constitutional weaknesses, cellular damage derived from infections suffered by earlier generations, and environmental pollution. This results from the mother's smoking habits, alcohol consumption, drug consumption and the stress factors she encounters during the first three months of pregnancy.

A prenatal causal factor in a patient suffering from recurrent cystitis may be an anatomical distortion of the opening of the urethra, a tethering of the urethra by the vestigial remains of a hymen (see page 42), or an inherited tendency to bladder neck dysfunction.

Postnatal factors include poisons derived from the external environment (lead in the atmosphere, mercury in dental amalgam, radiation, synthetic chemicals in processed foods), stress, physical injury and an inadequate diet. Causative factors derived from the individual's internal environment include allergies, disturbed intestinal bacteria following a course of antibiotics, and recurrent infections.

The 'mesotrophic' cellular decline resulting from the above factors is believed to come about as a result of the accumulation of toxic substances. These are derived from both the sources mentioned above, from diseased cells, bacteria and viruses, and from the metabolic processes of the body's cells. The toxins are regarded as collecting within the connective tissue or 'mesenchyme', the unstructured tissue surrounding the various organs.

It is through this substance that dissolved nutrients have to filter to reach the organs, and through which toxins have to filter to be eliminated by the circulatory system and the lymphatic system. Under normal conditions, elimination is finally carried out by the lungs (carbon dioxide), the skin (toxins dissolved in sweat and secreted on to the skin surface), the bowels (in the faecal waste) and the kidneys (in the urine).

When the mesenchyme is no longer able to store further toxic substances, and is deprived of necessary nutrients, saturation level is reached and what is known as the 'excretory phase' occurs. This is a sign that the body is attempting to rid itself of the gathering toxins, and typical manifestations at this stage are head colds, catarrh, diarrhoea, skin rashes and vaginal discharge.

Suppression of these by drugs (which is often the aim of conventional medical treatment) is, naturopaths feel, the cause of the condition developing into the next stage, namely the 'depositary'. This is typified by the formation of excretory phenomena such as the tophi (lumps) found in gout; arthritic nodules; fatty lumps ('lipomata'); and the fatty deposition within the walls of arteries (atheroma, which causes hardening of the arteries).

These, in turn, if not adequately treated by natural methods, lead to serious disorders which do succeed in overpowering the body's homoeostatic mechanisms, namely cancer, arthritis, multiple sclerosis, strokes, heart attacks, irreversible arterial disease and various serious mental disorders.

Because of the capacity of toxins to harm the individual, great importance is attached to the normal functioning of the eliminatory systems. The natural roughage of a wholefood diet with a high content of raw fruit and vegetables aids the intestinal eliminatory functions; and skin, lungs and kidneys are encouraged in their waste disposal activities by means of skin brushing (see page 66), deep breathing exercises and the regulation of fluid intake.

The function of the RES (reticulo-endothelial system) is also of great importance to the body's capacity to resist disease. The RES refers to tissues throughout the body (in the spleen, bone marrow, lymph nodes) which produce defence chemicals capable of neutralizing bacteria and unhealthy cells, just as the white blood cells engulf and destroy invading bacteria. When waste is failing to be cleared adequately by the body, the RES first becomes more active than usual, then starts to fail in its attempt as the burden grows too great.

This is referred to as a state of 'tissue uncleanliness', and is worsened by the added accumulation of toxins derived from the external environment (see page 57). It is this condition which naturopaths believe account for much of the 'generally unwell' feeling many people experience, without being able to point with precision to any one particular set of symptoms.

Regarding infection, naturopaths do not regard this as resulting from the invasion of a perfectly healthy organism by pathogenic (disease-causing) bacteria and viruses. Many of the micro-organisms (collective term for these two entities) that are responsible for disease succeed, at other times, in living within their host organism (human being, animal, plant) without causing it any harm.

Naturopaths in fact attribute the succumbing of an individual to pathogenic effects to the 'fault' of the individual, due to a change in the equilibrium of his internal environment. We return at this stage to contemplate the three vital factors upon which this equilibrium depends, i.e. structural, biochemical and emotional.

Because they see infection primarily as a sign of inner dysfunction, naturopaths do not generally advocate the use of antibiotics for the treatment of infection. This is a moot point about which more will be said in the final chapter; but the naturopath approach to treating disease – in particular, cystitis and urethritis – will be looked at in this chapter.

Diagnosis
Naturopaths take a case history and usually carry out a physical examination in much the same way as that used by your GP. The naturopath is likely to ask you more questions about your lifestyle, though, regarding stress factors, ability to relax, type of exercise taken and your diet. This is because, in addition to the urinary symptoms which caused you to consult him in the first place, he sets out to establish your overall energy level, and your ability to cope with factors that threaten your health. Your build and physical 'type', for instance, are important from a naturopathic point of view, certain bodily characteristics tending to be associated with a number of common disorders.

Further questions with which you would not be faced in your GP's surgery, and which may seem pointless to you at the time, could include whether you prefer raw food to cooked, warm air to a cold breeze, or certain colours to certain others. The answers to such questions give the practitioner useful information from the naturopathic point of view, in that they reveal important aspects of your make-up and your overall vitality.

Case history questions will very likely be aimed, also, at revealing possible prenatal as well as postnatal factors that might have contributed to your condition. The practitioner will ask questions about the health and lifestyle of your parents and grandparents, past medical conditions, treatment received and your response to them, and the time of onset and the duration of your present trouble.

A single cystitis attack, of recent origin, for instance, might be seen in the light of an attempt at toxic elimination on behalf of the body, or as a healthy response to pathogenic organisms or to chemical irritants. A long history of recurrent urinary problems, on the other hand, would more likely be seen as attempts by the body to cleanse the system which have failed because of interference from antibiotic drugs.

Many naturopaths use similar diagnostic tools to those employed by conventional practitioners. X-rays, blood tests and – certainly in your case – urine analysis would be likely. In addition, though, a naturopath may use supplementary methods of diagnosis to complete the picture he requires of your energy levels and overall vitality.

Iridology may be one of the supplementary techniques. In this, close examination of the iris of the eye for signs of significant hereditary traits, such as kidney or bladder weakness in your case; inherent constitutional stamina; and degree of toxic encumbrance in various parts of the body – in your case, possibly affecting the elimination of waste by the kidneys.

Another form of supplementary diagnosis might be *hair mineral analysis*. You are likely to have heard of this, as a number of articles have appeared about it in the Press, some of which have extolled its virtues and others of which have described it as inaccurate and useless. A considerable amount of research, money and effort have been put into establishing its value, and it is now becoming recognized as a useful adjunct in many instances to overall nutritional assessment.

A sample of head (or body) hair is used, weighing in the region of a few grams. A sophisticated laboratory technique known as spectroscopy is used to determine the levels of most of the major nutritional minerals, such as iron, calcium, magnesium, sodium and potassium, as well as of certain trace elements known to be significant in the maintenance of health, such as selenium, zinc and vanadium.

Care and experience have to be exercised in the final interpretation of the results. High or low levels of a number of minerals do not necessarily reflect an excess or a deficiency of that mineral in the body, and the readings following spectroscopy are considered in close conjunction with the dietary intake of the subject. All the same, the levels obtained are considered to be a useful indication of many of the body's minerals.

An example of body mineral levels possibly relevant to your cystitis attack is the condition of 'hypercalcaemia', in which the blood level of calcium is abnormally high. Hair mineral analysis is not in fact usually used as an indicator of the body's calcium status, as high levels in the hair can, in fact, mean that too much is being excreted, and that the level in the blood is low rather than high.

Nevertheless, when the level of calcium in the blood is raised, cystitis may be one of the results, since this causes an increased output of calcium by the kidneys, and this in turn can lead to the formation of kidney and bladder stones (calculi) and subsequent infected urine.

Radionics is another diagnostic technique a naturopath might employ. This is based on the understanding that bodily products such as a hair sample, urine, blood or saliva radiate the energy vibrations of the person from whom they were taken. A sample (known as the 'witness') is taken (it can even be sent by post), and is placed by the practitioner in a 'black box' which concentrates the energy field and enables him to tune in to those vibrations.

The particular application of radionics in which a naturopath might be especially interested, is the diagnosis of food sensitivities, organ vitality, toxic tissue accumulation and infective foci. Any of these might be relevant to a cystitis sufferer.

Radionics is also used as a form of therapy, appropriate corrections in the subject's energy levels being made by means of the 'black box'.

Naturopathic treatment

The methods used by a naturopath in treating any disease are aimed at increasing the patient's 'functional capacity', i.e. his ability to overcome the unbalancing effect of harmful stimuli. The detailed case history he had taken, combined with his physical examination, urine tests and the results of alternative diagnostic investigations, would have provided your naturopath with a good idea of your functional capacity and vital energy, and this would help him to decide upon the approach he should adopt in treating you. He would also know whether your cystitis symptoms were due to bacterial infection or to an irritant of another kind, and this would also be a decisive factor in the treatment.

Fasting and diet

You may have associated naturopathy, in the past, with the
imposition of fasting periods, followed by the stringent re-
organization of diet. Naturopaths do prescribe fasts where these
are appropriate, i.e. where the vital reserve, or reserve of energy,
is high, and the individual is likely to benefit from this measure.
But many, if not most, naturopaths nowadays are opposed to the
idea of radical treatment at all costs, especially where the cost
concerned involves what little energy reserve their patient still
possesses.

You have, basically, to be fairly fit in a general sense to
withstand and benefit from fasting. It is an age-old method well
deserving of its excellent reputation in ridding the body of
unwanted toxins, resting the digestive tract after perhaps a lifetime
of abuse and neglect, and stimulating the body's healing powers.
Fasting, which is essentially the voluntary abstention from food,
may consist of taking nothing other than mineral water, or freshly
squeezed fruit or vegetable juice, or be modified to include a little
of one particular type of fruit.

Fasting in one form or another is prescribed by naturopaths for
a wide range of disorders ranging from febrile illnesses (childhood
fevers, influenza) to acute conditions such as gastro-enteritis, and
rheumatism, and chronic ailments such as mucoid colitis, and chest
conditions. Whether or not you were prescribed several days of
fasting, would depend very much upon the extent to which you
had become debilitated, and whether you were receiving
naturopathic treatment by visiting a practitioner's consulting
rooms, or in a clinic in which you were resident for a few days.

Whatever the cause of your cystitis, it is highly likely that a
wholefood diet would be prescribed. We will go into the details of
wholefood eating in the final chapter dealing with the total self-
help programme; but it is essential to mention here how much
importance naturopathic and other alternative practitioners attach
to a wholesome diet.

Processed foods, and any dietary items containing synthetic
chemicals, from orange squash to the coloured icing on cakes, the
additives in factory-made, plastic-wrapped 'brown bread', and the
chemistry lab flavouring and preservatives in prepacked freezer
convenience meals, would be banned. And a definite emphasis

would be placed upon complex carbohydrates (real wholemeal bread, cereals, grains and pulses), raw foods in salads and desserts, and health-restoring items such as fresh, live yogurt, fresh fish, lightly steamed vegetables and the occasional free-range egg.

Tea and coffee consumption would be very greatly reduced and ultimately stopped, and you would be encouraged to substitute herbal teas, mineral water, and freshly squeezed fruit and vegetable juices.

If you were suffering from a cystitis attack at the time of your consultation with the naturopath, he would without doubt urge you to leave alcohol, coffee, tea and cola drinks well alone until you had recovered. He would also advise you about the proportions of acid-making and alkali-making food items in your daily eating habits, and probably provide you with a list of the two main varieties.

No naturopath would expect you to make all these changes overnight. It is no light matter to change a lifetime's eating habits, and you would be shown how to introduce the changes gradually, both for your own sake and for the sake of others for whom you cook! Nevertheless, as an immediate measure in treating your recurrent cystitis, you would be advised to alter some of your habits right away.

These would include eliminating from your diet all those irritants I mentioned earlier as possibly causing urethritis through irritation, and any foods to which you were sensitive. A method quite commonly employed by alternative practitioners nowadays to determine whether their patients are sensitive to any dietary items, is that of 'applied kinesiology', which you may have heard referred to as 'touch for health'.

Applied kinesiology is both a diagnostic and a therapeutic system, and a naturopath would either be experienced in it himself or would refer you to a specialist. Reduced to very simple terms, it is a system based on special muscle-testing techniques through which weaknesses are identified and treated and imbalances in the body's energy systems corrected. By means of applying special diagnostic tests, a professional kinesiotherapist can detect a food allergy or sensitivity response in a patient's muscle groups, and pinpoint which food items are very likely responsible for unwanted reactions – in your case, recurrent cystitis or urethritis attacks.

Elimination of toxins

Of great relevance to your current balance of vital energy, especially when this has been depleted by recurrent attacks of infective cystitis and prolonged antibiotic treatment, is the degree of saturation of your tissues with toxic waste. A common sequence of events in these circumstances is that your body tissues reach a considerable degree of 'uncleanliness' (toxin saturation – see page 57), and this depletes your vital reserve of energy.

You then are unfortunate enough to pick up a bacterial bladder infection, and have insufficient resistance to deal with it. You succumb, develop symptoms and your GP treats you with an antibiotic. Fair enough, so far as orthodox reasoning is concerned, but if your lifestyle does not counteract the depleting effects of the drug therapy and of the toxin accumulation upon your defence mechanisms, then the problem will clearly recur. Each attack further depletes your energy reserve, and makes subsequent attacks more and more likely – and less and less easy to get rid of.

There are several methods your naturopathic practitioner might employ to generate healing, marshall your innate defence mechanisms against invading bacteria, and restore unstable energy balances. But in naturopathic practice, toxin elimination remains one of the most important.

We have seen that a fasting period (generally lasting between three and seven days), followed by changes to wholefood eating, can be very useful in this respect. Another manner in which whole foods, containing natural roughage or fibre, is helpful is in the formation of regular, bulky stools which help to keep the large bowel free from the toxin-producing, stagnating contents often found in people on an 'average' diet, which is high in refined foods and synthetic substances and low in bulk.

Besides large bowel elimination, your body will be encouraged to reject toxic accumulation through your skin, lungs and kidneys. Your practitioner would know, from his physical examination of your spine, joints, tendons and muscles what degree of structural imbalance existed, and also what type of exercise would be best suited to your needs.

It is commonplace today to find people suffering from far too little exercise, with resultant muscular tension, skeletal aches and pains, and sore, stiff joints. If this applies to you, you would be recommended to become gradually accustomed to stretching, bending and moving harmoniously, perhaps through the medium of dance therapy or yoga, and then when you were sufficiently fit, to start on a gradually progressive programme of aerobic exercise.

Postural problems and structural imbalance would be corrected as and where necessary, and the perspiration produced during aerobic exercise would effectively remove some of the toxic waste stored within your tissues.

The lungs as eliminatory organs
Exercise, in whatever form you were advised to take it, would definitely improve your breathing! Not until you were at the stage of fitness where you could exercise aerobically, would a physiological demand by your tissue cells for more oxygen be actually made upon your heart and lungs. But dance therapy, involving free expression and simple bodily movement to music under the guidance of a trained teacher, would indisputably get you taking long, deep breaths in harmony with whatever movement you were performing; and yoga is renowned for improving mental, physical and spiritual balance and stamina, not least by the emphasis it places upon learning to breathe properly.

You may feel that you breathe perfectly adequately, since you never suffer from coughs or chest problems, and that only people who suffer from asthma or chronic bronchitis require advice about breathing. Nothing could be further from the truth, in fact, because very few of us who are not trained to use our lungs to their optimal capacity, utilize anything like the full potential they have to offer.

If you think of the degree of lung power Sebastian Coe, Mikhail Baryshnykov or Harry Secombe must have developed, you will have a clearer idea of what wonderful organs the human lungs actually are. These three stars are not 'special' anatomically; they started off in life much the same as you or me as regards their breathing capacities. But they learned, early on, to use their respiratory systems to their greatest advantage, to serve them in their chosen roles.

You may not wish to run, dance or sing professionally. But you definitely wish for a healthy life, and the lungs are perfectly adapted to provide you with the most important of biochemical requirements, oxygen. As their capacity for supplying oxygen to your blood improves, you will find that your own subjective experience of energy and vitality improves, not to mention a general improvement in your body's overall vital force.

Part of this beneficial effect is due to the greater supply of oxygen your blood now carries, and part of it is due to your increased elimination of the toxic waste, carbon dioxide. Practise your deep breathing out in the open, as far away as possible from atmospheric contamination, and you will also be aiding your body in its perpetual battle against airborne pollutants such as lead, sulphur dioxide and other industrial by-products.

Elimination through the skin
Besides the excretion of toxins in sweat, there is another method by which naturopaths encourage the elimination of toxic material through the skin. The rate of toxin disposal increases enormously during a fasting period, and when you are eating a diet containing a high proportion of raw fruit and vegetables such as described in the best selling book on 'high-raw' eating, *Raw Energy*, by Leslie and Susannah Kenton (Century Publishers). It is likely to be under these conditions that the technique of skin brushing would be most beneficial.

This consists of speeding up toxic waste loss (up to a third of the body's wastes can be eliminated through the skin) by brushing your entire body surface, apart from your face, with a rough hemp glove or a long-handled natural bristle brush.[6] You start at your feet, and brush from the soles upwards, up both legs, front and back, with sweeping strokes. You then brush the rest of you, reaching your back by stretching with the glove or by means of the long-handled brush, using a firmer touch all over but a little more gentle on your abdomen (where the movement should be clockwise), chest and neck.

The authors of the book from which I am quoting, then suggest a warm shower, followed by a thirty-second cold one. Incidentally, the naturopathic technique of skin brushing speeds up the disappearance of cellulite, the thick, bumpy fat layer often found disfiguring the thighs, bottoms and upper arms of many of us who have less than perfect figures. This is especially true when it is combined with a high-raw diet, as also does aerobic exercise.

Waste elimination through the kidneys

Everyone knows that the kidneys play an enormously important part in the elimination of toxic wastes from the body – as they do, of course, in maintaining our bodies in a suitable state of fluid balance and in regulating the acid-alkali balance within the blood. Failure to excrete waste toxins satisfactorily is one of the main reasons why many people with diseased kidneys depend upon kidney dialysis machines to stay alive.

Without the use of such a machine (or a successful renal transplant), these unfortunate people would actually die from poisoning by their own toxic waste – in particular, urea, a breakdown product of protein metabolism. This fact indicates only too clearly the importance of properly functioning kidneys.

It is a standard procedure to tell people suffering from cystitis attacks, bacterial or irritant, to drink large quantities of fluids. This 'flushes out the kidneys' (which actually means that the kidneys are provided with a larger volume of water than usual into which to secrete the toxic materials they have filtered off from the blood, which in turn has collected from the rest of the body).

Toxins have to be in solution in the blood-stream before the kidney tubules can filter them off efficiently and then reabsorb some of the water, thus forming urine. And a 'dialysis', an increased output of water by the kidneys, enables this to happen.

The other, more obvious way in which large quantities of fluid are extremely useful in cystitis, is in flushing out the bladder and urethra. Any bacteria multiplying in the bladder or ascending the urethra will tend to get swept back down in the urine stream the more often you urinate. A very dilute urine, preferably alkaline in reaction, is far less painful to the inflamed lining membrane of the lower urinary tract. And chemical irritants will be disposed of more rapidly as well.

Emotional balance

We have seen, in the course of this chapter, the different approaches a naturopathic practitioner would take to solving the problem of your cystitis. These 'different approaches' are, in fact, all inseparable parts of the application of naturopathic theory to the far greater underlying problem of poor energy reserve.

We have seen how he would help you to make dietary

alterations gradually over a period of time, and how to adopt an exercise routine which would correct postural strain, restore you to a state of physical fitness and enable you soon to include an aerobic exercise regimen into your lifestyle.

We have also seen the attention he would pay to your eliminatory mechanisms, namely the lungs, skin and kidneys. In all these ways, two of the basic factors upon which vital energy depends, the biochemical and the structural, would have been reinvigorated and brought into closer harmony with one another.

There only remains to mention the attention your naturopath would pay to your mental and spiritual elements. This may *sound* very nebulous, but in fact is a vital part of the overall treatment, and an aspect of management that many orthodox doctors today tend to neglect.

Your case history would have revealed details both of the stresses to which you are normally subject, and your reaction to them. On the strength of these findings, he may suggest changes in lifestyle that would mean less stress, and also, very probably, he would point out the wisdom of learning how to relax properly, either from instructions he would give you himself, or from a tape or book, or from a psychotherapist or hypnotherapist.

The techniques involved in the learning of adequate relaxation are discussed in Chapter 9, which deals with psychotherapy and hypnotherapy.

Many naturopaths employ the professional skill of other alternative therapists to aid the healing process. Alternatively, they may possess other skills themselves which, besides applied kinesiology, might include qualifications in herbal medicine, homoeopathy, acupuncture or perhaps aromatherapy. Applied kinesiology has been referred to as the 'fastest growing alternative therapy in this country' and your naturapathic consultant might very well utilize the techniques involved for their therapeutic energy balancing powers, as well as for their diagnostic potential.

6

Herbal Medicine

The use of plants as remedies is certainly as old as civilization, and almost certainly older. Records dating back to around 3,000 years BC list plants valued in both China and Egypt for their medicinal properties, together with the ailments to which they were applicable. In this country, herbs are used in three main fields of alternative medicine – medical herbalism, aromatherapy and Bach flower remedies.

Herbal medicine
It is fairly certain that our early ancestors chose herbs by means of an instinctual awareness of their healing properties. Both wild and domesticated animals exercise this ability today, when allowed to roam freely. And in the earliest times, herbal medicine and magic were inextricable, formalized ritual being an essential element in much of the selection, gathering, preparation and administration of plant remedies.

Later, although the use of plants in magical ritual continues today, as sources of incense, perfume, hallucinatory effects, mental stimulation and increased sexual vigour, plants gradually came to be used as sources of medicine which could be applied without attendant ritual and ceremony. All the same, their astrological correspondences are still regarded by some modern herbalists as an important aspect of their use, and many organic gardeners recommend the planting and gathering of vegetables and herbs at certain times in the moon's monthly cycle.

However fascinating this information may be, you are doubtless wondering quite what all this has to do with your cystitis attack. If there *are* herbal preparations that can be used to relieve pain on passing urine, the need to make frequent visits to the toilet, blood and perhaps pus in your urine and a low, dull back or stomach pain, why do I not write down their names immediately and explain where to obtain them and how to use them?

I shall certainly be providing these details further on in this chapter, but it is essential, first of all, to show you how medical herbalism 'ties in' with the holistic medical principles discussed at length in the previous two chapters. Many people think that taking a preparation of feverfew for a migraine attack, for example, or a cup of sage tea for its calming effects, is much the same as taking a couple of paracetamol, or some valium! In other words, that herbal preparations are no more than the crank's equivalent of an efficient drug.

Of course herbal medicine offers a number of symptomatic remedies for a variety of ills, and these are available for anyone to purchase either from a medical herbalist or from a health food store. Better still, if you have the time, interest and opportunity to do so, you can identify which herbs you need to form a herbal remedy, discover where they grow, and gather them and prepare it for yourself.

Despite the numerous herbal medicaments available, though, the theory of herbal medicine is essentially founded upon holistic principles, or perhaps it is more accurate to say that it developed from the instinctual practice of holism by our remote ancestors, when the intuitive faculties now vestigial in us, were a vital element of Man's successful relationship with his environment.

Herbal medicine has many advocates among satisfied patients in this country. It ranked as the most popular alternative therapy, according to a major survey involving 2,000 people, commissioned by Swan House Special Events, backed by Newman Turner Publications, in 1984. Twelve per cent of people questioned had tried herbal medicine, and 73 per cent of them had found it satisfactory.

Theory
Herbal medicine recognizes the presence of 'vital force' or 'vital energy' and, like naturopathy, pays tribute to its inherent powers of self-correction and self-healing. Again like naturopathy, herbal

medicine sets as its task the identification of elements of weakness within an individual's total energy field, followed by the treatment of any weaknesses detected by the restorative and balancing effects of plants.

Symptoms are seen as a useful indicator of their underlying cause, and it is this that constitutes the focal point of the medical herbalist's attention. Disorders are believed to arise only in potentially unhealthy individuals whose tissues permit the development of pathology by being 'unclean' due to poor circulation and the accumulation of toxins.

The presence of a stone in the kidney or ureter, for example, would be regarded as the equivalent of the naturopathic 'depository' phase, in which the body is losing its battle to get rid of waste material accretion. Ureteric colic, caused by a large renal stone getting stuck within the hollow of one of the ureters, and the resultant smooth muscle spasm which tries to squeeze the stone down into the bladder, would be viewed as the combination of an irritant factor, and a tendency to strong reactions.

The infective aspect of bacterial cystitis would be seen as an indication of 'stagnation' in the tissues of the bladder and urethra, permitting bacteria to flourish; and the inflammatory aspect of irritant cystitis attributed to a healthy but inadequate attempt by the body to get rid of toxic accumulation.

There are three main ways in which herbal medicines act.[7] The first of these is by *toxic elimination*, and the preparations a medical herbalist would select would usually be backed up by advice about a wholefood diet which also encourages the disposal of toxic waste. Like that recommended by the naturopath, it would contain a high proportion of raw fruit and vegetables and freshly squeezed fruit and vegetable juice.

Herbal medicines can aid elimination by their effect upon the sweat glands, lungs, bowels and kidneys. This reduces the overall tissue uncleanliness of the patient and improves his supply of vital energy. Examples of eliminatory herbs include angelica root, elder flowers, yarrow, camomile and pennyroyal which promote perspiration; butternut root, dandelion and senna, which promote elimination from the large bowel; and diuretic herbs.

Diuretic herbs increase the output of urine (and therefore of excretory products) by the kidneys. This is a desirable effect in cystitis, where increased urine output not only gets rid of extra toxins but also increases the rate at which bacteria are washed down the urinary tract and out via the urethra (I mentioned earlier their tendency to climb the ureters and reach the kidneys).

A bonus of diuretic treatment in cases of cystitis, whether or not bacteria are the cause, is the very dilute urine formed. Since diuretic herbs are not being prescribed in your case to get rid of accumulated body water (water-logged tissues have many causes, such as the premenstrual syndrome, kidney failure and heart disease, but not uncomplicated cystitis), you will of course be asked to drink larger volumes of than usual of water and juice. Dilute urine is far less painful to pass than small volumes of highly concentrated urine, and this in itself will help to relieve the pain.

Examples of diuretic herbs include parsley root and leaves, feverfew, meadowsweet, borage and garlic.

In addition to encouraging elimination, herbs can often be chosen *to protect* the body in some way, and bring about a specific healing activity. Just as the naturopath aims at evoking the body's natural and innate self-restorative powers, by the application of natural stimuli such as water, fresh air, sunlight and a natural diet, so the medical herbalist seeks to do the same with his choice of herbs.

A practical application of this is seen in the use of herbs that protect the body in some way, giving relief from symptoms, and then proceed by virtue of this protection, to set the healing process into motion. An example is the use of aloe vera juice or gel to an ulcer or area of burned skin. This substance has a soothing and anti-inflammatory effect on damaged tissues and mucous membranes, and this in turn encourages healing to occur. (Not all inflammation, however, is beneficial. Although I pointed out in Chapter 1 that the inflammatory reaction is a healthy defence mechanism upon which we depend, chronic inflammation as found at an ulcer site or associated with a burn injury, is of limited value and needs to be counteracted before the healing process can be completed).

An example of a herb used in cystitis for its anti-inflammatory (and thereby health-promoting) effect, is marshmallow root. This has a calming, anti-inflammatory effect upon a painfully inflamed bladder and urethral lining membrane, and helps it to regain its normal healthy condition.

Health food shops often sell the powdered root. My recommendation is to add a third of a pint of boiling water to a heaped teaspoonful, and to stir it until a gelatinous mixture is formed. Leave it for ten minutes and then take it before eating. This should be carried out three times a day during and immediately after a cystitis attack.

The use of diuretic agents in cystitis is also, incidentally, an example of triggering a healing reaction by means of appropriate herbs.

Thirdly, many herbs help restore a body organ and ultimately the body as a whole, to normal function, by supplying certain nutrient ingredients that their isolated active constituents or their synthetic equivalents could not supply. This action can be loosely summarized by saying that the whole plant (or part of a plant, such as its roots, petals or bark) fulfils a greater number of the body's needs and supports its health in more ways than the sum of its individual parts would be capable of.

The word for this effect is 'synergism'. The zoological and botanical worlds show countless instances of synergism, and it is believed to be due to the component parts of a system in some way potentiating one another's actions so that the system works far more effectively as a whole (or whole part of an) organism than just the total of its individual parts.

Often a really useful herb has dual, or multiple, mutually complementary activities, attributable to its mixture of complex active constituents. Couchgrass is an example. This herb is used for its properties as a diuretic, and for its ability to calm pain due to inflammation and spasm in the urinary tract. It also contains an antibiotic substance called agropyrene, a form of antibacterial agent which will not upset your helpful intestinal flora, and therefore will not cause diarrhoea, flatulence and possibly thrush infection.

Couchgrass might be prescribed for you in the form of its dried root, the dose being 1-4g three times daily or more often if advised. Other herbs with urinary antiseptic properties your medical herbalist might choose for you, include golden rod, shepherd's purse and celery seed.

Aromatherapy

Aromatherapy consists of the use of natural plant and herb essences for healing purposes. These essential oils are complex aromatic (i.e. scented) compounds, many of which have been analysed by modern scientific methods and whose range has been made more accessible by modern distillation methods. Despite the useful intervention of modern technology, however, much remains unknown about how these plant essences achieve their curative effects.

The art of aromatherapy extends back in time to ancient China, Egypt and India. Aromatic woods and resins were burned to purify the air, the antiseptic properties of precious oils and aromatic gums and spices (all plant products) were used to prevent dead bodies of revered rulers and sacred animals from putrefying, during the process of mummification, and scented oils and plant essences were massaged into the skin both to relieve the strained muscles of wrestlers and charioteers and to keep early facial wrinkles at bay.

At one time, a major aspect of the use of aromatic oils was their therapeutic effect upon the senses, via the sense of smell. Now, 'aromatherapy' refers more extensively to the curative benefits to be achieved by administering these oils in such a way that their biologically active constituents are absorbed into the bloodstream and the body tissues. Aromatic essences are, therefore, now capable of being massaged into the skin, into which they are generally transported by a 'carrier' oil in which they are soluble, such as ultra-pure, cold-pressed olive, peanut or sweet almond oil; alternatively, they might be massaged into the skin in a carrier wax (such as beeswax) or a fat.

They can also be taken by mouth as an alcohol preparation, as an emulsion in water, or as a few drops on a little brown sugar or honey; dissolved or emulsified in wine or cider vinegar; and inhaled in steam.

There are around 200 essential oils extracted on a commercial basis.[8] Of these, about sixty have well-recognized therapeutic properties and are commonly used in aromatherapy. Besides being taken by mouth or applied to the skin as a massage or rub, essential oils can also under certain conditions be injected, or administered as a bath, a compress, a douche or an enema.

When given by mouth, the majority of the essential oil is excreted via the urinary system, usually in combination with a substance called glucuronic acid which the kidneys often use for the purpose of 'carrying' excretory substances out of the body in the urine. This makes aromatherapeutic remedies an excellent form of alternative or supplementary treatment for disorders of the kidneys, ureters, bladder or urethra, since these are brought into intimate contact with the chosen essence.

Many aromatic essences might be mentioned in connection with the kidneys and urinary tract. Rosemary essence stimulates and tones up several vital organs, including the kidneys; lavender essence has a wide-ranging anti-bacterial effect, and rose essence (also known as 'Rose Otto') acts primarily upon the liver, kidneys, stomach, heart and, most especially, upon the female reproductive organs.

Essence of cajeput (Melaleuca Leucodendron) is often recommended for cystitis. The essence is inhaled, often twice daily, and five drops of the essence are taken on a little brown sugar three times daily.

Bach flower remedies

The 'Bach flower remedies' consist of thirty-eight carefully prepared remedies derived from flowers and are particularly interesting because they are designed to remedy negative emotional states rather than to act directly on physical disorders. They were invented by Doctor Edward Bach, a qualified medical doctor who at one time practised as a pathologist and bacteriologist at University College Hospital, London.

Edward Bach became dissatisfied with orthodox medicine and studied homoeopathy. The emphasis in homoeopathic medicine upon the patient and his or her individual temperament and emotional make-up, rather than upon their symptoms, led him in the direction of the beliefs upon which he later founded his own system of medicine. His theory was that emotional problems and negative thought patterns are the underlying cause of physical disorders, and that the best way to remedy the latter was to correct imbalanced attitudes in the former.

Homoeopathic practitioners use much plant-derived material, and Bach, seeing how efficacious homoeopathic treatment can be, sought among plants and their flowers for his own materia medica.

Using his considerable intuitive powers, Bach derived his thirty-eight remedies from wild flowers whose qualities he was able to pick up by testing their effect upon himself. In order to capture their ethereal curative qualities, the flowers are treated precisely according to a prescribed ritual, and this method is never deviated from even today, fifty years after his death. The flower heads are placed on the surface of water, preferably spring or well water but never distilled water, in a plain glass bowl and left in full sunlight for three hours. The resultant liquid is strained, preserved by the addition of an equal volume of brandy, and labelled 'basic stock'.

This is diluted in the proportion of five drops of the stock to one fluid ounce of water, and it is then bottled.

Edward Bach claimed that his remedies worked because they possessed the power to 'elevate our vibrations, and thus draw down spiritual power, which cleanses mind and body, and heals'. His system of medicine is holistic in principle, since it recognizes the vital interplay between the intellectual, physical and spiritual elements of our nature, and seeks to remedy disorders through aiding disordered emotions.

He is also clearly referring to our electromagnetic field, vital energy and life force, when he speaks of our 'vibrations'. He differs only in that he seeks to draw down the life force of the universe as the necessary element in curing imbalance, rather than attempting to stimulate the body's own innate healing powers.

These remedies are especially applicable to people with negative emotions. Most long-term or recurrent disorders can sap our sense of vitality and pleasure in life, and cystitis is particularly adept at inducing the kind of hopelessness that feels there never will be an end to the repeated bouts of unpleasant symptoms.

Which remedy would prove most appropriate for you, would depend upon your emotional make-up. Few Bach flower practitioners exist, but the remedies can be obtained direct from the Bach centre, Wallingford, Oxford, or from health centres. Especially recommended for 'despondency and despair', are the following remedies: larch, pine, elm, willow, sweet chestnut and star of Bethlehem.

7

Homoeopathy

I mentioned at the end of the last chapter how Doctor Edward Bach became so fascinated by the concepts of homoeopathy that he abandoned his pathology career and studied that system of medicine instead. His action was even braver (some would say more misguided or foolhardy!) then than it would be now, for homoeopathic medicine was still regarded by many of his contemporaries as unscientific and nonsensical, and the law forbade its practice by anyone not already qualified in conventional medicine.

Homoeopathy has, however, proved its efficacy time and again in the treatment of many diseases, and it is now valued by many people, including some orthodox doctors and millions of grateful patients, as an acceptable, if puzzling, alternative to conventional medicine. Not only does it achieve the ends for which it is prescribed; it has the great advantage over drug therapy of not producing side-effects.

Homoeopathic remedies are, in fact, very gentle and entirely non-toxic, and one of the stimuli to its development by Dr Samuel Hahnemann during the eighteenth century was the crudeness and violence of some of the methods orthodox medicine then employed. Purging and bleeding (often for the very disorders we now recognize as being the least suited to these methods) were everyday practices; and suitable care for the mentally sick, the retarded and the emotionally disturbed was non-existent.

The simple-minded but harmless petty thief was incarcerated in a hellish 'bedlam' of a lunatic asylum, side by side with violent paranoid schizophrenics and misguided young girls who had had the misfortune to become pregnant once too often without finding a husband. Orthodox medicine has made enormous strides over the past 200 years, and we have a great deal for which to thank modern medical research. But looking back at the conditions that prevailed when homoeopathy came into being, it is easy to see the reasons why more humane (and successful) methods of treating patients were sought.

What, you are probably asking at this point, has all this got to do with cystitis? Again, I suggest that it is better to know a little about any form of treatment before deciding to accept it for oneself. Those who know even less than 'a little' about homoeopathy, still sneer at the apparently contradictory concept of 'potentizing by dilution' – as indeed I have puzzled over it myself in the past. You can obtain homoeopathic remedies for yourself from a chemist or health food shop; or consult a homoeopathic practitioner if your cystitis symptoms are not relieved by self-help measures and simple remedies. Either way round, you are likely to seek help more quickly if you are convinced that homoeopathy has something concrete to offer you. And time is of the essence in dealing with cystitis attacks.

Dr John Clarke, a famous homoeopathic physician who died in the early thirties, called homoeopathy: 'The most complete and scientific system of medicine the world has ever seen.' Many practitioners subscribe to this view. But this is not to say that homoepathy can be used in every single instance, and is capable of acting as a substitute for surgery, for specialist care in, say orthopaedic medicine or obstetrics, or for the detailed clinical investigations of complex disorders.

None of the disciplines – not even orthodox medicine – is capable of solving every medical problem; and the best and most experienced practitioners in every field know when to draw the line and refer their patients elsewhere. Infected kidneys (pyelonephritis), as I have stressed elsewhere in this book, constitute a potentially life-threatening condition and immediate investigations followed by antibiotic treatment is at present the best treatment available.

A tendency to form renal or bladder stones (calculi) however, and recurrent infective or irritative cystitis and urethritis, can be treated very effectively by homoeopathy, and may well obviate the need for you to take – to no avail – yet another antibiotic course.

Theory

Samuel Hahnemann was particularly interested in biochemistry, and besides treating patients as an orthodox doctor, he carried out experiments into the nature of drugs. One of the methods he adopted, was to try out the effect of drugs designed to cure a variety of disorders upon himself when he was *not* ill.

The drug that particularly took hold of Hahnemann's imagination was quinine, used overseas to treat malaria and introduced into Europe by travellers from those areas where malaria was rife. He discovered that a dose of quinine produced in him those very symptoms that a malaria patient in need of quinine would experience. It made him feel weak, toxic and feverish, and he deduced from these effects that the symptoms of malaria do not constitute the actual disease, but are the form taken by the body in its attempt to overcome malaria.

Investigating other drugs along similar lines, and using both himself and healthy volunteers as guinea-pigs, Dr Hahnemann discovered that the same rule applied. It then seemed more logical to him, to encourage the body in its attempts to remain healthy by administering doses of a compound that produced the same 'symptoms' in a healthy person, than to adopt the approach of orthodox medicine, which does its best to damp down the symptoms of disease as soon as they arise.

Does that mean, in your case, that taking a homoeopathic remedy for cystitis symptoms, would give you worse pain on passing urine, increase its content of blood and pus, and increase the number of your night-time visits to the loo? Cystitis symptoms, in common with the symptoms of any other disorder treated homoeopathically, might be very slightly exacerbated for a short spell shortly after your course of treatment started. But relief would be highly likely to follow a short time afterwards.

The principle serving as the foundation stone of homoeopathy is that of: 'like cures like'. Samuel Hahnemann was not the first to enunciate it. The physicians of Hippocratic Greece were aware of its truth, and the idea flourished once again for a brief time during the Renaissance.[9] Moreover, doctors during the century preceding Hahnemann's, were taught by the great physician Thomas Sydenham that the symptoms of a disorder were an indication of the body's fight to resist disease processes. This latter idea accords closely with the naturopathic view of the symptoms of acute disorders that we looked at in Chapter 5. The principle of 'like curing like' also forms the basis of vaccination (immunization) in which a tiny quantity of the disease-causing organism or its toxin, is injected into the body to prevent an actual attack of the disorder concerned.

The use of tiny quantities is also an essential aspect of homoeopathic medicine. In the thirty years preceding the publication of his book: *Organum of Rational Healing* in 1810, Hahnemann continued his detailed observation of the effects of drugs, and he discovered to his surprise that diluting a compound by shaking it up in water *increased* its potency instead of *decreasing* it.

He called this process of dilution 'succussion' or 'potentization', and soon proceeded to make his medications more and more dilute or, in his own terms, more and more powerful.

He went from potencies of 1 in 100 to 1 in 1,000 and greater, finally reaching the 30th potency, and performing all his succussion by hand. Finally, of course, it was impossible that a single molecule of the original compound could still remain in the solvent carrier (it is now known that there is no physical substance left after about the 12th potency).

Nevertheless, practical experience confirmed for him, time and again, that homoeopathic medicaments were indeed at their most potent when thus diluted. Other medical practitioners strongly disapproved, though. Innovative ideas in any walk of life seldom appeal to other practitioners of the same profession or discipline who have *not* thought of the idea before. The fact that they are successful, has little effect upon the strong prejudice that arises against the concept's inventor, except, of course, to strengthen that prejudice and increase the extent to which others feel threatened.

Hahnemann was laughed at as a fool, and prosecuted for endangering the livelihood of the rest of the medical profession. He was forbidden to practise by an Austrian court, and returned to his laboratory investigations at Leipzig. However, he was returned to favour when he treated a member of the royal family successfully, and was permitted to practise once more.

Six editions of Hahnemann's *Organum* appeared in all, and in the later editions we see the philosophy that goes hand in hand with the theory and practice of homoeopathic medicine. He had always maintained that medicine should aid the body in its attempts to resist illness, and this way of thinking developed over the years into a more complete picture of the body's vital force. He recognized that this 'vital force' was identical with life itself, and his most mature view of it was in close agreement with that of naturopathic practitioners.

Like them, he maintained that it was the life force that empowered an organism to gain ascendency over the onslaught of a disease process, by the exercise of innate forces within that organism that sought always to rectify energy imbalances within it. The foundation of homoeopathic thought was, therefore, established upon sound holistic principles, and Hahnemann recognized the supreme significance of the patient as an individual, whose state both in sickness and in health is a manifestation of personality, physical constitution, spiritual well-being and intellectual and emotional make-up.

The actual symptoms which bring a patient to a homoeopath, therefore, are but one aspect of the case that interests the practitioner. As each individual is different, two people with the same symptoms, e.g. a burning sensation on passing water, with blood in the urine and getting up three times nightly to empty the bladder, may require completely different treatment. You, for instance, may have a pale complexion, auburn hair, a love of the colour green and a dislike of cold drinks, whereas a friend or relative may be ten years younger than you, have straight, fair hair, be allergic to mushrooms and suffer from claustrophobia. All these facts – and many others – are enquired about during the initial consultation, to enable the homoeopath to form the kind of picture of his patient that he needs in order to decide upon the most appropriate remedy.

Treatment
Quite frequently, patients comment after receiving homoeopathic treatment that they feel a great deal more energetic than they have for a long time. Part of the reason is the rebalancing and harmonizing effect that homoeopathic medicine has had upon their vital force. Part, too, is the fact that energy-sapping experiences such as a recent bereavement, repressed anger or

jealousy, the loss of a job or a possession, a law suit or the termination of an emotional relationship, are asked about and taken into consideration during the case history. These causes for ill health can all be dealt with effectively by the administration of the appropriate remedy.

Homoeopathic remedies may take up to several weeks to work. There may be, as I mentioned earlier, an aggravation of the symptoms by the remedy used, and these may become more intense until they finally disappear. It is considered to be good and correct homoeopathic practice to encourage the patient to bear with the treatment until the irritation phase is overcome and energy balances have been successfully restored, at which point the symptoms will have disappeared, often for good.

It is not considered competent practice to resort to a second high potency within a few days or a couple of weeks of the first prescription to alleviate the discomfort of the exacerbation. Patients who receive several high potency preparations in rapid succession often suffer from extreme nervous disturbance and excitement, and this is believed to result from there being too many powerful energies in the body at one and the same time.

Homoeopathic remedies likely to be prescribed for cystitis include Cantharides (which is Spanish Flies, often written as 'CANTH'); Staphisagria (which is Stavesacre, often written as 'STAPH'); and Causticum ('CAUS'), which is Tincture Acris Sine Kali.

Cantharides is one of the commonest medications to be prescribed for bladder conditions. Indications for its use in patients with cystitis symptoms are the presence of burning when urine is passed, together with urgency, pain after urine has been passed, blood in the urine, and pain associated with urination in the bladder itself or in the urethra.

Added indications confirming the likelihood of Cantharides being useful, are the worsening of symptoms while urine is actually being passed, and after drinking cold water.

Staphisagria is typically prescribed for 'honeymoon cystitis', when contributory factors to the condition are likely to include bacterial contamination from the anal region, possibly some bruising of the urethral outlet as a result of frequent intercourse, again possibly the introduction of a little dirt, dust, sand granules from the husband's fingernails, and – also possibly – over-indulgence in alcohol, strong coffee and tea!

Further irritant factors are likely to include all the pleasantly scented toiletry the bride takes away with her, from talcum powder, bath essence and scented soap to perfumed vaginal deodorants, bubble bath liquid and nourishing oil for her skin.

Concomitant factors which point to Staphisagria as the choice of remedy include worsening of the symptoms after taking cold drinks, the symptoms being worse in the morning, sensitivity to emotional hurt, the vagina feeling painful due to pressure from clothes, improvement of the symptoms when warmth is applied, and feelings of dissatisfaction regardless of what comfort or remedies are offered.

Causticum is perhaps less likely to be the remedy of choice for young patients with cystitis, but can prove very useful in older women. The particular indication for its use is leaking of the urine in the form that we call 'stress incontinence' because it occurs following coughing or sneezing. These are not precisely forms of stress as the word is generally understood, but they both cause the muscles forming the front wall of the abdomen to be contracted, with a resultant momentary increase in the intra-abdominal pressure and consequently in the intra-pelvic pressure too.

A bladder whose neck has become slightly weakened, may well be further irritated by infection and inflammation and the added strain may prove too much for it. A number of reasons exist for a weak bladder neck. Some women seem to have a tendency to the condition, and this is aggravated by, perhaps, slight prolapse resulting from several years of child-bearing, carrying heavy weights (such as the weekly shopping, and small children), or fibroids in the womb. Other predisposing factors include being overweight, perhaps a chronic (smoker's?) cough, a diet poor in fibre and bulk, and chronic constipation.

Slight urinary incontinence can also follow pelvic operations on the bladder, urethra or womb, and it is usually quite easy to rectify surgically. However, when it occurs in conjunction with cystitis, it is an indication for the suitability of Causticum.

Other indications for this remedy include a feeling of anger before periods start, or melancholy (severe depression) experienced during this time.

8

Acupuncture and Acupressure

So far, with the exception of naturopathy, the alternative forms of treatment we have looked at, have been aimed primarily at rectifying energy imbalances at the biochemical level (see page 56). Of course, since both herbal medicine and homoeopathy are based upon the principles of holism, both seek – as much as does naturopathy – to bring all three elements of body, mind and spirit into harmonious balance. They achieve this both through the herbal and homoeopathic remedies their practitioners prescribe, and by the advice the latter give their patients about exercise, relaxation, their emotional welfare, and, where applicable, their spiritual needs as well.

Nevertheless, neither professional herbalists nor homoeopathic specialists would object to my saying that the means each adopts to achieve his ends is primarily through alterations in energy at the biochemical level.

In this chapter, we are going to look at two holistic therapies that may be of use to you as a cystitis sufferer, and that are aimed at rectifying energy imbalances at a structural level. In the next chapter we will see what contributions psychotherapy and relaxation methods can make to your total well-being.

Acupuncture

I mentioned earlier, in discussing evidence for the existence of vital energy, that the Chinese refer to this factor as 'Ch'i', and that it is to impediments to its free flow throughout the body that they attribute disease. I also explained that, since scientific evidence has now been obtained for the existence of meridian lines and acupuncture points, acupuncture as a form of therapy has become more credible to the Western mind and has gained acceptance with orthodox medical doctors.

While all thinking people must applaud the wider acceptance of a form of therapy that has been practised for thousands of years – one, in fact, that represents a most effective weapon in dealing with pain and disease – I feel that we doctors as a professional body have made too rapid a 'volte-face' in the following respect. One minute, it seems, medical science regards acupuncture as nonsense, and those who practise it as fools and charlatans, but then it is said that scientific methods have proved that vital energy, meridian lines and acupuncture points *do* exist, and controlled acupuncture trials have shown that excellent results can be achieved. Acupuncture has been granted a 'clean bill of health' and, furthermore, doctors proclaim that only medically qualified practitioners should be permitted to practise it!

Obviously, as a doctor myself, I cannot help sharing many orthodox views with my colleagues (remember how I stress the necessity for proper investigation into the cause of your cystitis, and for antibiotic treatment for the infective variety), but I can see no reason whatever to deny non-medically qualified acupuncturists the right to practise. Clearly, all therapists, whatever their calling, need proper training; and properly trained and qualified acupuncturists are the first to acknowledge this need. Charlatans and 'learn-acupuncture-in-one-weekend' therapists need to be weeded out, for the sake both of prospective patients and of acupuncturists who have studied this therapy for a long time.

Acupuncturists, however, were carrying out safe and effective treatments for thousands of years before we as a profession deigned to study their speciality. And I cannot agree that suddenly, after all this time, it has become unsafe to allow non-medically trained members of their profession to continue to do so.

Experienced acupuncturists are aware of the types of disorders that are likely to be improved by their treatment; and are usually quite ready to suggest full medical investigations and additional or substitutional orthodox treatment where this is applicable. To suggest that they (trained acupuncturists) do not know when to withhold treatment and when to seek further opinion, is to suggest that they are both ignorant and irresponsible.

It has also been suggested, with reference to the philosophy upon which acupuncture is based, that 'it is not necessary to believe in folklore to understand and accept acupuncture . . . there is now sufficient knowledge available for acupuncture to be taught and practised as an exact, objective technical discipline, but this status has not been achieved in the UK because it is still firmly based on the traditional approach'.[10]

With this view, I am only in partial agreement. Granted that it is possible to practise acupuncture successfully, without possessing a detailed knowledge of ancient Chinese beliefs, I feel still that we dismiss the wisdom of the ancients, supplanting it by 'exact, objective technical discipline', at our peril. The practice of medicine was an art, relying upon a mixture of instinctual awareness and intuitive deduction, long before it became a science, and a great many centuries before 'technical disciplines' were heard of. Demand a scientific basis for every aspect of the healing arts, and dismiss the underlying beliefs as 'folklore', and one arrives at a bastard practice from which the essential kernel – the understanding of the hidden aspects of Man's nature – has been ruthlessly torn.

Theory
Acupuncture is holistic in its approach, aiming at balancing and freeing the patient's energy flow and not simply at the relief of symptoms. (It can be, and often is, used to relieve troublesome symptoms, including pain, especially when used as an adjunct either to orthodox medical treatment or to another alternative therapy, but acupuncturists generally much prefer, wherever possible, to correct the underlying disorder).

The Chinese concept of Ch'i shares much with the Western naturopathic concept of 'vital energy' or 'life force', in that it is the essential element present in all living things, and lacking in dead, decaying ones. While naturopathic philosophy readily concedes the presence of the 'life force' throughout the whole of the natural world (some hold that it is present in 'non-living' objects such as earth, stone, minerals, water and air), it does deal primarily with its existence within Man.

Eastern philosophy, on the other hand, takes as much cognizance of the life force on a universal scale as it does of that share of it that each of us individually possesses. As a system it is all-embracing, seeking to harmonize Man's inner being (and thereby his health and vitality) with that of the universe in which he lives. Ch'i is, moreover, the motivating force behind and within the universe, and expresses itself in two mutually complementary modalities, called Yin and Yang.

Yin and Yang are present in all matter, the proportion of one to the other depending upon the nature of that invested matter. Yin characteristics are those that are traditionally associated with femininity – softness, penetrability, negativity, flexibility, mildness. Yang qualities are the opposite, and traditionally masculine in nature – hardness, penetration, positivity, inflexibility, aggressiveness.

Ch'i enters the body at birth, and flows around it in a harmonious fashion all the time the person is in a state of health. Its flow is directed along certain paths (meridians), which the Chinese insist are not the same as nerves, lymphatic pathways or blood vessels and cannot be equated with any physical structure however much Westerners try to rationalize them. The flow of Ch'i along these meridians is not constant but, in a manner comparable to the ebb and flow of the ocean tide, varies in harmony with the changing pattern of the universe.

It is affected by the weather, the seasons of the year, the time of the day or night, and Yin and Yang are in a perpetual state of fluctuation. For a person to be healthy, these two qualities have to be in a state of balance, i.e. in the correct proportion to one another throughout the body; they do not have actually to be present in equal amounts. When a person is sick, there is an excess of either Yin or Yang somewhere in his energy system. The insertion of needles at specific points along the meridian channels, corrects the disproportion and relieves the disorder.

Also taken into consideration is the link between the five elements, fire, metal, water, earth and wood, which are produced by Yin and Yang, and the organs with which these are linked – the heart, lungs, kidneys, spleen and liver respectively. These are 'solid' organs and are Yin by nature. Each is affiliated with a 'hollow' (Yang) organ, which again respectively are the small intestine, the large intestine, the bladder, the stomach and the gall-bladder. The existence of two further organs, unknown to Western doctors, is recognized. Both are Yang by nature, and the first is called the 'Triple Warmer', while the second is known as 'The Gate of Life'.

Physiology, or the working of the body, is described and interpreted in terms of the interaction of the elements, the seasons, and the associated organs. Summer, for instance, is linked with fire (for obvious reasons), and therefore with the heart. Just as the seasons develop successively, and just as the the elements interact (water destroys fire, for instance) so by parallel association can the kidneys cause heart disorders. These are merely a few of the factors an acupuncturist has to pay mental attention to when you ask him to treat your cystitis.

The acupuncture points are situated along the course of the meridians, each of which is primarily either Yin or Yang by nature. The kidney meridian, for example, is Yin, and it runs from the sole of the foot, up the leg and abdomen to the chest. The bladder meridian is Yang; it starts on the nose, runs upwards over the top of the head, and down the back of the chest, abdomen and pelvis to the leg, to end on the last joint of the large toe.

In all, twelve chief meridians are recognized, as well as a number of subsidiary ones. They have variable numbers of acupuncture points associated with them – for example, there are sixty-seven along the course of the bladder meridian. Well-trained acupuncturists, of course, take into consideration the nature of the symptoms of which their patients are complaining, and are aware that certain meridians and acupuncture points are thereby loosely indicated. But, as mentioned before, of equal importance to his final choice of acupuncture points, is whether Yin or Yang predominates at the time of consultation, in that particular season and in association with the particular weather conditions that predominate.

Deciding whether the quality of Yin or that of Yang is greatest in strength under the prevailing conditions, and determining where the imbalance lies, enables the therapist to decide which quality to tranquillize and which to stimulate.

Diagnosis is made largely by means of pulse palpation (feeling the pulse). This takes an acupuncturist a great deal longer to carry out than it does an orthodox doctor, because six pulses in each wrist have to be examined, one for each meridian. On the left wrist, for example, three superficial pulses are first felt for along the length of the radial artery near the wrist – these provide information about the small intestine, gall-bladder and bladder, and urethra.

The three deep pulses on the left wrist, indicate the state of energy balance within the heart, liver and kidneys.[11] In addition to feeling these twelve pulses, the acupuncturist claims to pick up details of twenty-seven different qualities in each of them, each giving valuable information about a specific disease. For this reason, while examination of the pulses throughout the body may take an orthodox specialist five to ten minutes – to assess thoroughly the condition of the entire circulatory system, arterial pulsation at wrists, elbows, neck, abdomen, groins, knees (deep within the hollow of the joint, felt from behind with the patient's leg flexed at the knee), and ankles (in front and behind, where the two main arteries enter the foot), and the rise and fall of pressure waves within the jugular vein – pulse assessment by an acupuncturist may take up to two and a half hours.

Besides this method, the acupuncturist also notes certain things about his patient, such as texture, condition and colour of the hair and skin, the brightness or dullness in his eyes and the smell of his body odour and breath, the timbre of his voice, and the condition of his tongue. The tongue, for example, gives information about the urinary system, particularly the kidneys.

Treatment

Having obtained as much information as he needs, the acupuncturist will then weigh up all the evidence and decide in favour of one or several sites at which to insert his needles. This is either painless, or very mildly uncomfortable, and the therapist has a choice of nine different needle types. The ones which might be applicable to you, are the 'spoon' needle (if you have strong pulses), the stiletto needle (if your cystitis is chronic), and the round, sharp needle to relieve pain.

Having decided whether to stimulate or to calm Yin or Yang within a chosen meridian, the acupuncturist takes his chosen needle and either inserts it hot, or cold, depending upon whether Yin or Yang is to receive attention. For Yin, cold needles are chosen, and for Yang, hot. If the chosen element is to be stimulated, the needle is inserted with speed and withdrawn slowly. It is rotated in a clockwise direction to stimulate Yang, and anticlockwise to stimulate Yin. The pulses are felt with the needle in place, and withdrawn when the therapist feels it is the right moment.

The area of insertion is massaged gently with the fingertips after the needle has been withdrawn. If Yin or Yang is to be quietened, then the procedure is the same as just described, but the area is not massaged afterwards.

Whether you need one treatment or several, or one every so often at regular intervals, will depend upon how quickly you take to respond satisfactorily.

Acupressure

Another technique an acupuncturist might either try (if you are really very scared of needles) or might tell you about so that you can practise it at home when necessary, is acupressure. This is a method for applying treatment at acupuncture points by finger pressure instead of by needle insertion, and while it does not have the specificity of action or the finesse of the needle technique, nevertheless, very desirable results can be obtained with it, simply and painlessly.

Acupressure can in fact be used to relieve a variety of problems (travel sickness, for example; a 'problem' appetite, when you are trying to diet; and dental pain are only three of them). In your case, it could be very valuable for you to have an additional drug-free, natural, pain-relieving method quite literally at your finger tips, to deal with a painful cystitis or urethritis attack should you suffer another.

The area to which to apply finger pressure to relieve acute pain is on the upper lip, in the midline, midway between the root of the nose and the top of the 'lipstick' area. Press lightly at first and you will know where your particular point is because you will feel a definite pain sensation there as a result of pressure, whereas this will be missing only a millimetre or two away from this point in any direction.

Lie down or sit down quietly away from any sources of disturbance and massage the area gently with your forefinger pad, using a light circular clockwise movement, and rotating the skin against the underlying upper jaw bone. Continue this for between one and five minutes. Subsequently, you can try stronger pressure on this spot with your forefinger nail, applying pressure for ten second intervals and releasing for ten seconds in between. Again, this is performed for between one and five minutes.

You can do this as many times a day as it is necessary and there are no side-effects.

For chronic pain, locate a point on the back of either hand, about three of your own finger breadths below the gap between the fourth and fifth fingers. Apply light persistent pressure here, always with the ball of the forefinger of the other hand, as described above for acute pain relief. The instruction is normally given to remember to choose the point which lies on the same side of the body as the pain, but this is unlikely to apply to either cystitis or to urethritis pain.

All the same, this point might come in useful if you are unlucky enough for infection to ascend to one or other of your kidneys.

9

Relaxation and Hypnotherapy

In this chapter we are going to see how hypnotherapy may be able to help you to overcome cystitis. Hypnotherapy is, of course, a type of psychotherapy, and I feel that I must explain exactly why I have chosen to include it. My reason for wishing to make this clear right from the start of the chapter is that some readers may perhaps feel as some patients do when the GP – unable to cure them to their satisfaction – in desperation (or so it seems to them) suggests an appointment with a psychiatrist.

This is sometimes enough to prevent a very sensitive patient from returning to the surgery for a long time, so incensed does she (or he) feel by the implication that her disorder is 'all in the mind'. This is a pity, since the GP is often misunderstood on this score. It is not *only* holistic philosophy – it is a universally accepted fact – that the mind is inseparably integrated with the body, and orthodox doctors are coming to realize more and more nowadays that there is little advantage in ignoring the one and treating the other.

Sometimes, of course, family doctors do diagnose a particular patient as hypochondriacal, or as having an underlying depressive illness, or clinically recognizable anxiety, and very little wrong with them physically. Very frequently, though, they recognize that the patient's physical symptoms are only too real (i.e. a barium meal reveals a peptic ulcer, perhaps, or cystoscopy shows an inflamed bladder lining), but still feel that these physical changes are generated by anxiety. This is not at all the same thing as implying that they are imaginary. Pent-up anxiety stemming, for instance, from emotional problems in infancy or early childhood, or from excessive amounts of stress over a long period of time, is known to cause actual physical changes in a person, generally attacking the particular system that has shown a weakness in the past.

It is only by getting to the root of the problem, weeding it out, and helping the patient to start afresh and equipped to cope with problems, that doctors can be of help. There is nothing to be gained, apart from very temporary relief, from giving remedies for troublesome symptoms alone. This is why I am suggesting that hypnotherapy might prove a very useful adjunct to your overall plan to free yourself for life from cystitis attacks.

If you decide to rely entirely upon self-help measures (once your urine has been tested and any initial bacterial infection treated – see final chapter), you may decide to find a hypnotherapist for yourself. This you can do by consulting your GP, by looking through Yellow Pages, or by personal referral from someone who is already a patient.

You might, on the other hand, be referred to a hypnotherapist after first consulting a naturopath. He or she will, as I explained in Chapter 5, be aiming at restoring your energy levels from the three main viewpoints of your biochemical state, your structural condition and your spiritual-emotional well-being. If you are usually a happy, relaxed and carefree sort of person, not at all prone to depression or anxiety, then he may simply discuss your lifestyle with you to discover whether you are being subject to any specific psychological or emotional stress that may be contributing to your your cystitis attacks.

If he detects, though, that you are depressed, angry, resentful, and basically pretty anxious, then he is likely to suggest some form of psychotherapy that he feels might be of use to you.

Anxiety
It is worth deciding what exactly anxiety is, and how it can harm us – in particular, how it might help to cause cystitis symptoms – before looking at what hypnotherapy is, and how it works. Once you have insight into the meaning and implications of the anxiety state, you will be far better able to decide what part, if any, this condition plays in your health problems.

Everybody is familiar with the word 'anxiety'. You may describe yourself as feeling anxious about your husband who is late home from work, anxious that your children will do well at school, anxious about how you are going to make ends meet, and – yes, very anxious about your recurrent cystitis symptoms. But when doctors and psychotherapists use the word anxiety, they draw a clear dividing line between two closely associated conditions – anxiety and worry.

You may feel that they are identical; but technically, worry refers to feelings of concern *about* a particular person or situation, and anxiety refers to feelings of concern that are sufficiently strong to cause discomfort and apprehension, yet cannot be related to any particular circumstance in the mind of the subject.

Now, worry is bad enough. It is dreadful to fear that your housekeeping, temper or health – or all three – are going to give out before the end of the week, and you naturally worry about the difficult shopping, the rows, or the visit to your doctor's surgery that will be the inevitable result. But at least, if you approach them the right way, you can do something about these matters. Knowing what is troubling you, is half way to solving the problem, even if the solution is far from ideal in your own eyes.

Anxiety, on the other hand, is diabolical. It is a very common condition, and there is no hope of relieving it by taking appropriate action. It arises in many of us for a whole host of reasons, but the one I mentioned earlier in this chapter, emotional disturbance in early childhood, deserves a few words of explanation.

Freud and his followers identify three stages of psychological development. The first two, the 'oral' and the 'anal' stages, take place during infancy and need not concern us here, apart from mentioning that they are believed, when impeded by child-parent conflicts, to provide the foundations for depressive illness, the schizoid personality, schizophrenia and other mental disturbances later in life.

Conflicts during the third, or 'genital' stage, however, are capable of setting the scene for the development of anxiety neurosis later on, in individuals who are naturally susceptible to this condition, and who experience other predisposing problems and conflicts during the course of their maturation. Also called the 'phallic-oedipal' phase, the genital stage starts when the child is about three years old and is characterized by the child's increasing interest in his or her genitals, together with a tendency to worry about, and/or ask questions about, the physical sexual differences between the two genders.

I say 'a tendency to worry about' – as well as to express curiosity about – sexual affairs at this infantile level advisedly. Certainly, it would be unusual for a baby or toddler to be predisposed to 'worry' from birth (maybe there is a gene that transmits a worrying personality, but I haven't personally heard of it). But small children *can* nevertheless feel anxious and guilty about sexual matters even before they enter the true genital phase, if their experiences during babyhood have laid the foundations for these feelings.

Factors predisposing to an anxious personality during babyhood, might well be present in the attitude of one or both parents to their own and their baby's sexuality, although it is highly unlikely that either the mother or the father would be aware that anything was amiss.

You may not believe that babies and small children are affected by the small details of attitude and behaviour that constitute the emotional background of their family life. But babies whose small hands are instantly removed from 'down below' if they happen to touch their genital areas from curiosity or boredom; whose parents never kiss, caress and cuddle one another in his sight; and who generally adopt a severe and restrictive attitude to anything resembling sexual playfulness, *are* more liable to repress innocent questions and self-exploratory experiments and to worry inwardly, when they come to the genital stage.

It is often an extension of this parental behaviour towards and in front of the child, from birth and throughout childhood that, from the age of three years onwards, causes real damage to the child's psyche. The injury results from the transformation of genuine if embryonic sexual feeling into one of guilt, and from three onwards to the age of five or six is the most likely time for this to happen, since it is during those years that the toddler becomes aware of 'attraction' to the parent of the opposite gender to himself (hence the term 'oedipal' as used above).

This is a normal phase through which all babies pass, and one that is, of itself, capable of generating guilt and anxiety (due to being torn between pleasing and winning one parent, and possibly incurring the wrath of, and retribution from, the other). If this phase is badly handled, and the child has already been introduced to an infantile awareness of guilt almost from the moment of birth, then psychological problems are bound to result that will express themselves in one or two ways later on. The first of these is the development of an hysterical illness, and this need not concern us here. The second is the development of an anxiety neurosis.

The name Freud gave to the anxiety experienced by someone suffering from this condition, was 'free floating'. It is constantly present (even if occluded for some of the time by other matters demanding attention), and flavours all other experiences to a greater or lesser extent with the acrid taste of apprehensiveness, fear and hopelessness. People who are persistently anxious rarely enjoy anything to the full –particularly not sex – and sexual difficulties, frigidity, impotence, vaginismus (difficulty of penetration due to tightly clenched vaginal and pelvic muscles) are common problems.

The physical symptoms caused by anxiety can be very distressing. These include a dry mouth, a racing pulse, unpleasant churning sensations in the stomach, and frequently the need to open the bowels or spend pennies more often than most other people. Ultimately, free-floating anxiety and its accompanying physical symptoms give rise to a full-blown 'panic' or 'anxiety' attack, and it is often after experiencing one of these for the first time that the anxiety sufferer will visit his or her doctor.

Parallels have been drawn between this experience and the sexual act, and it is easy to see why. The physico-emotional energy that mounts and overspills during such an attack, is very similar to the mounting excitement, energy and tension that ascends to the peak of climax during sexual intercourse, and then subsides after it has discharged itself. The heartbeat increases in speed and volume; the breathing becomes heavy and rapid; the pupils of the eyes dilate, the mouth dries, one's hair feels as though it were standing on end, and the muscles go stiff and rigid.

Whereas intercourse and climax are a highly pleasurable experience, though, the panic attack is terrifying and exceptionally unpleasant. The sufferer feels 'terrified' without knowing of what, and all the vague disquietude and apprehension he has grown almost used to as an everyday occurrence, seem suddenly justified by the imminent arrival of his ultimate doom.

The damage anxiety attacks can do, however, can be even more serious. The energy crescendo of the initial attack carves memory patterns in the subconscious mind and affects the individual's autonomic nervous system and glands responsible for producing the physical effects. This makes subsequent attacks more and more likely, and at the same time anxiety is inextricably bound up with sexual feeling and expression.

Of greater relevance to you as a cystitis sufferer, though, if you *are* suffering from neurotic anxiety and panic attacks, is that the mind needs, and has to find, something to which to attach its intolerable free-floating anxiety. There are three possibilities – the development of a phobia, the 'externalization and identification' of the anxiety into concern for the welfare of others, and by the development of physical symptoms.

Bodily symptoms are always experienced during a panic attack, and they frequently hit hard by adversely affecting the body's weakest system. If, in your case, this is your bladder and urethra, then these are likely to become the focal point at which future symptoms are manifest, in a 'symbolic' manner, to provide your mind with an 'explanation' for the anxiety you experience. When bout after bout of mind-generated bladder or urethral problems have been experienced over a period of months or years, actual physical changes occur, producing in some cases a demonstrable urinary problem, weakness of the bladder neck, difficulty, perhaps, in emptying the bladder completely at any one time, and a consequent tendency both to contract urinary infections and to suffer persistent urethral irritation.

Theory of hypnotherapy

Although the human mind is extremely complex, the theory upon which hypnotherapeutic treatment is based is fairly simple. The mind is divided into two regions, the subconscious (unconscious) and the conscious. The subconscious mind is the repository of every single memory of every single event that has ever happened to us, both pleasant and unpleasant. Its contents are set free when we dream and can be reached when we are in a trance state, induced by hypnosis, and when we are half-asleep, dozing between true sleep and wakefulness.

The conscious mind is the part we think, reason, feel and plan with – the faculty with which we are consciously aware of ourselves and our surroundings on a minute-by-minute basis. Situations and events we 'take in' consciously, are passed down to the subconscious region where a memory tracing of them is formed, and where they are stored for future reference. That future reference may be by means of our conscious mind, which has no problem in recalling from the subconscious region, millions of facts which it needs for its daily functioning.

Future reference may be difficult, however, and only be available when steps are taken by an analyst or hypnotherapist deliberately to investigate a particular repressed (hidden from conscious recall) fact. Thoughts and feelings, and certain memories, are deliberately repressed by the subconscious mind, if they have proved injurious and painful, and – so far as it is concerned in its protective role – better not disclosed.

Unpleasant thoughts and feelings, even if generated many years ago, however, can continue to cause damage to the psyche at a subconscious level. It is by these means that babyhood conflict and early guilt experience can succeed in engendering anxiety neurosis at a much later stage in life.

I have said that the contents of the subconscious mind can be reached during hypnotic trance. This is the purpose of inducing such trances, i.e. to contact the patient's subconscious storehouse of forgotten memories and discover the underlying reason for the build-up of anxiety and tension. This is usually possible; and when it is, realization of the 'reasons why' is often very therapeutic, if not curative, in itself.

When the initial childhood problem cannot be recalled even under hypnosis (the memory may be too well hidden in the subconscious, or so painful that the patient unwittingly resists its revelation), therapeutic suggestions can still be made successfully while the patient is in a state of trance which will gradually loosen the bonds by which anxiety neurosis is binding him.

Once he is free from free-floating anxiety, he becomes free from its attendant symptoms and the need for other physical problems to which to attach that anxiety. This gives disorders such as recurrent cystitis and urethritis, and symptoms such as 'frequency' (frequent need to pass water) and 'nocturia' (getting up in the night to pass water) the chance to clear up in response to appropriate treatment.

Neither hypnotherapy, nor the majority of the other forms of psychotherapy, are comparable to naturopathy in their approach. Hypnotherapeutic theory does not speak of 'vital energy' or 'vital force', nor does the practice of the art take account of tissue toxification, structural problems, or the biochemical nutritional status of the patient. Nevertheless, the aim of hypnotherapy is to identify and reveal the underlying cause of the problem, since it views this as the only way to achieve lasting results; hence its proper practice is in no way aimed at symptomatic relief only (except in special circumstances where pain relief may be all that can be done for a patient).

Moreover, it attaches much importance to the interaction between mind and body, and the importance of treating a patient bearing both in mind. Hypnotherapy is neither a true orthodox therapy, nor a true alternative one. It lies on the dividing line between, and may be seen, perhaps, as a valuable bridge or meeting point between the two of them.

Treatment
A hypnotherapist starts a consultation by taking a case history. He would be interested in your present symptoms, past complaints both physical and emotional, past treatments, past injuries, shocks and traumatic events, and – probably – details of your childhood, parents, brothers, sisters and family life.

Instead of carrying out a physical examination, he would then test your suggestibility. One way is to suggest to you that your arm is getting lighter and lighter and rising without your making any effort. This works in some people, not in others.

He might also test your degree of trust in him, by getting you to stand in front of him with your back towards him. You would be asked to let yourself 'fall' backwards into his hands, as he is standing close behind you. Most people can let themselves go in the required way; others cannot.

He would then check that you were comfortable, and didn't need to visit the loo or remove a jacket or coat. He would settle you down in an easy chair or on a couch and set the lights low or draw the curtains.

You would then be asked to close your eyes and count backwards from, say, three hundred to one, concentrating on what you were doing and not consciously listening to his suggestions. While you were thus engaged he would start suggesting that you were growing more and more relaxed, more and more sleepy, heavy, floppy and tired. The actual words, and the actual induction method, have many different forms. But essentially the therapist is getting you to use (distract) your conscious mind while he gains access to your subconscious.

Monotonously repeated suggestions made in a congenially relaxed setting, while your conscious mind is engaged in other activities that demand its concentration, make it possible for the therapist to reach your subconscious regions. Thus, by suggesting that you are getting more and more relaxed, he succeeds in inducing a light state of trance.

When this has taken place, you will feel comfortable, relaxed, dreamy, yet aware of his voice. You are likely to feel warm, and your arms and legs and body perhaps, pleasantly heavy and tingly. In addition, muscles that are often tense such as those of the abdomen, the eyelids, the back of the neck and the tongue, feel relaxed and comfortable.

What exactly has happened is that – while your attention has been deliberately fixed elsewhere – the therapist's voice has been carried by specialized nervous pathways in the brain that normally deal with sound and thought. All other stimuli having been cut off, his voice alone is received and thus is able to overcome underlying anxiety, resentment, resistance and other negative emotions. It reaches its goal, your subconscious mind, and has direct access to your store of memories and repressed emotions.

He may then deepen your trance by, for instance, describing a scene in which you are standing at the top of a short slope or flight of steps, and down which his words gradually guide you, telling you as you 'go down' that your trance is deepening. When at the bottom, you are as deep as he intends you to go.

This account in fact summarizes the progress of several therapy sessions. During the first, the therapist and you may be content with a detailed discussion and a trial induction of light trance. As time goes on, however, the therapist will gain an idea of your underlying problem, and be able – say, by the third or even the second session – to suggest reasons for your underlying anxiety which he will have diagnosed in all probability from the first consultation.

He can gain further information from your subconscious mind about underlying causes in infancy, by getting you to signal 'yes' or 'no' by a pre-arranged finger movement. You may or may not remember his questions and your answers when you return from the trance state. If the recalling of some traumatic event causes you distress under hypnosis, this may have a very beneficial effect on your disorder. Alternatively, the therapist may feel that it would be a good idea to discuss after the trance state has been reversed, what your underlying problems really are.

Either way round, coming face to face with them is usually a healing experience, if rather traumatic at the time.

During the trance – and as soon as he has sufficient information – the therapist can give you a relaxation symbol to visualize each time you feel anxious between sessions. He will instruct you under hypnosis to picture your symbol – a rose, a candle flame – each time you feel symptoms coming on, while at the same time you take deep breaths and repeat, for example, 'peaceful and relaxed . . . peaceful and relaxed'.

This, he will assure your subconscious mind, will succeed in having the calming effect your anxiety symptoms need, and will eventually overcome them altogether. His instruction to you to do this, between sessions, together with assurance of the desired result, is called 'planting a post-hypnotic suggestion'.

You will probably be taught the art of relaxation; and very probably taught autohypnosis, so that you can encourage the speed of your recovery between sessions. I will go into autohypnosis as a self-help measure in the final chapter.

10

Self-help Measures

In this final, short chapter, I am going to sum up the self-help measures I have mentioned throughout the book, to make certain that you are armed with as much information as you need to bid cystitis a permanent 'farewell'.

1 Check-up
Next time you experience the warning signs that an attack is imminent, take a mid-stream urine specimen (MSU) and see your doctor. If he is used to sending specimens off for you anyway, ask him for a couple of proper sterile containers to have by you for when you need them – otherwise one never seems to have a small, empty screwtop jar in the house when a cystitis attack starts.

Whether your urine was tested last month, or has never been tested before, plase make sure that your GP sends the sample off, requesting 'microscopy, culture and sensitivity'. Take the antibiotic course he prescribes for you; better safe than sorry with bacterial infections and this will hopefully be the last you will need.

If you are a chronic sufferer from cystitis and/or urethritis, please get your doctor to perform an internal examination, plus a cervical and vaginal swab if there is any sign of infection. If you get recurrent infections and have never had the underlying cause identified, please request hospital investigations without delay (see Chapter 2).

2 Personal habits
Please re-read the advice I have given about contamination of the urethral area through the incorrect use of toilet paper, through sexual intercourse, through inadequate hygiene and through the

use of tampons. Discuss relevant points with your sexual partner, and make sure you wash your perineum before and after love-making, and that you open your bladder, also, after sex.

In particular:

* Avoid nylon panties and tights, tight trousers and jeans, all of which encourage sweating and maintain your perineal area in a warm, moist state, perfect for invading bacteria to multiply and flourish.

* Don't use the Pill, spermicidal cream, the cap or diaphragm, or let your partner use the sheath – at least until you have discovered whether avoiding these has any positive effect. You should try being without whichever one you normally use, for at least three months. An IUCD (intra-uterine contraceptive device) is probably the best in the meantime.

* Likewise, give up any use you may make of vibrators, or other sexual aids applied to the clitoris directly (because this is bound to affect the urethra as well). Apart from washing and drying the area – LEAVE IT ALONE! And avoid making love outside on a dusty, sandy or leafy surface, or with your partner unless he has scrupulously clean fingers and fingernails. You may sound obsessive, but it is you who has had, in the past, to put up with cystitis attacks.

* Avoid extremes of temperature – just do not be tempted to sit on cold stone walls or floors, or on radiators.

* Don't go swimming in chlorinated swimming baths. Try avoiding this for three months to see whether there is an improvement.

* Regarding your own bath-time habits, don't add antiseptic fluids, nor any scented, coloured or otherwise artificial product to your bath water. Only use plain, uncoloured and unperfumed soap, and avoid vaginal 'freshener' tissues and deodorant sprays.

* Avoid highly spiced foods, citrus fruit, pickles, citrus fruit juice and all alcohol apart from a really small 'social' glass on rare occasions. Avoid any foods to which you think you may have an allergy (and see page 21).

* Make sure you drink enough non-alcoholic fluid everyday to

replace that which you lose – and add 2 pt of bottled mineral water to this volume for good measure.

3 During an attack

When you have delivered your urine sample to your doctor and obtained a prescription from him, go home and go to bed! Get your prescription made up on the way home, take the course prescribed, get into bed with a hot water bottle to hold against your pelvis, and place a large 3 or 4 pt jug next to the bed (and a glass – you don't want any excuse for not actually drinking what you have put there!)

The jug should be filled with cold tap water, or bottled mineral water, and you should drink half a pint every half hour for three to four hours. Add 2 teaspoonsful of baking soda (bicarbonate of soda) to the first jug of fluid, or take this mixed with a little honey or molasses.

Take also a herbal diuretic preparation as described in Chapter 6. It is by far better to consult a medical herbalist personally. But if you are anxious to use a quick self-help measure, buy some Potter's Diuretabs from the nearest health food shop, and take two tablets three times a day, for three days, starting on the day your symptoms start. Keep up a good fluid intake during this time (you can relax from the half a pint every half hour routine a little, when symptoms have abated).

Take powdered marshmallow root three times daily for three days, as I have detailed on page 73.

You may, or may not, be able to get a couchgrass preparation from your health shop (see page 73). Again, it is best to see a medical herbalist who will select a urinary antiseptic for you personally. For a quick remedy of this kind, ask for dried celery seeds, golden rod or shepherd's purse, and infuse half a teaspoonful in a teacup of water for ten minutes, strain, reheat if necessary and drink three times daily.

Inhale some essence of cajeput (follow suppliers instructions about inhalation method) and take five drops three times daily on a little brown sugar.

Ask for a list of the Bach flower remedies from your health food shop and send off for the remedy you feel is most applicable to yourself.

4 Diet

If your symptoms persist despite all these measures, I suggest you go to visit a practitioner of one of the alternative therapies that I have already outlined. It is entirely up to you which type you choose, but a naturopath would seem to me to be a very good 'first' choice as his plan of campaign for your improved health is such a comprehensive one.

He will then, as I have mentioned, call upon other alternative practitioners to supplement his methods should this be necessary. I have given details of the type of diet a naturopath would select for you in Chapter 5. *Don't* cheat and drink alcohol, tea or coffee if he forbids it! And do avoid artificial additives in foods. You will be sure to find that you have far more energy and greatly improved all round health, after a period of three to four months.

5 Pain relief

For the relief of cystitis and urethritis pain, try the acupressure techniques I describe on pages 91–2. A medical herbalist will be able to give you a good pain-relieving herbal preparation if you wish to have one in preference to a pain-killing drug. I can personally recommend some herbal tablets named Tabritis which health food shops sell specifically for the pain and symptoms of cystitis. If you need to speed up the soothing effect of diuresis and marshmallow root, try these.

Autohypnosis

Lastly, I will mention how to relax and to use auto (or 'self') hypnosis, methods which are capable of transforming your life, let alone your health, if you will simply practise them in one twenty-minute session every day.

You are bound to be taught relaxation if you visit a hypnotherapist; and will probably be taught autohypnosis as well, as most therapists nowadays are anxious to equip their patients with self-help measures that will stand them in good stead – not just between sessions, but for the future, too.

Put aside a half hour in the day when you will be alone and undisturbed. You may have to wait until the children are in bed or your husband is watching his favourite TV programme – but work out the half hour of the day or evening you can call your own.

Sit or lie back in a comfortable chair, wearing loose and comfortable clothing, in a comfortably warm room that is dimly lit. Then settle down, and working up your body, starting with the muscles of first one foot and then the other, the muscles of one calf and then the other, clench and relax every muscle group in turn until you have covered all of them, including your scalp, eyelids and tongue, with which you should finish.

As you do so, say the words: 'Clench hard . . . and then relax . . . relax . . . . relax'. Wait a few seconds to feel how relaxed muscle groups *do* feel, then pass on up to the next group.

When you are relaxed all over (it is a wonderful feeling, especially after a stressful day, and it helps very much to have your eyes closed throughout the session), picture a symbol such as a flower or a candle flame, and count down backwards from ten to one. By doing this, and saying 'deeper, deeper', between each number, you will enter a light trance which will be useful for your purposes, but out of which you will, incidentally, awaken automatically, either if an emergency arises demanding your attention or if you accidentally go to sleep!

When you have got down to 'one', picture the inside of your bladder and urethra in an inflamed state (bright red, glistening and very tender), and when you can hold that image in your mind, spread a wave of cool blue healing light over the whole membrane, in your imagination, thus calming the inflamed nerve endings and removing the source of the pain.

Retain this 'whole', healthy new image replacing the old, angry inflamed one for at least five minutes. Then replace it with your flower, candle flame, whatever; contemplate that for a few moments; then count back up from one to ten again. Before you get up, shake yourself free, draw the curtains and put the kettle on (for a cup of *herbal* tea!), and tell yourself that whenever you feel a twinge of bladder or urethral discomfort in future (you may never!), you will picture your image of flower or flame. This will calm you down; and picturing your red inflamed membrane cells turning cool, healthy and non-irritant as the healing wave of blue light sweeps over them will remove the pain almost instantly, if you practise visualization every single day.

References

1. Hooper, Henrietta, *GP*, 17 May 1985, page 7.

2. Hooper, Henrietta, *GP*, 17 May 1985, page 7.

3. Swanson, Maureen, *GP*, 5 October 1984, page 37.

4. Potterton, David, *Doctor*, 5 May 1983, page 30.

5. Swanson, Maureen, *GP*, 5 October 1984, page 38.

6. Kenton, Leslie and Susannah, *Raw Energy* (Century Publishing, London 1984), page 113.

7. Fulder, Stephen, *The Handbook of Alternative Medicine* (Coronet Books, Hodder and Stoughton, 1984), pages 173-75.

8. Tisserand, Robert, *Journal of Alternative Medicine*, July 1984, page 15.

9. Inglis, Brian, and West, Ruth, *The Alternative Health Guide* (Michael Joseph Ltd., 1983), page 67.

10. Swanson, Maureen, *GP*, 5 October 1984, page 37.

11. Bartlett, E. G., *Healing Without Harm*, Paperfronts (Eliot Right Way Books), 1985, page 19.

Index